Health Essentials

Alexander Technique

Richard Brennan is a qualified teacher of the Alexander Technique, having completed a full time training course approved by the Society of Teachers of the Alexander Technique. He now runs courses and workshops, as well as giving individual lessons.

The Health Essentials Series

There is a growing number of people who find themselves attracted to holistic or alternative therapies and natural approaches to maintaining optimum health and vitality. The *Health Essentials* series is designed to help the newcomer by presenting high quality introductions to all the main complementary health subjects. Each book presents all the essential information on each therapy, explaining what it is, how it works and what it can do for the reader. Advice is also given, where possible, on how to begin using the therapy at home, together with comprehensive lists of courses and classes available worldwide.

The *Health Essentials* titles are all written by practising experts in their fields. Exceptionally clear and concise, each text is supported by attractive illustrations.

Series Medical Consultant
Dr John Cosh MD, FRCP

In the same series

Acupuncture by Peter Mole
Aromatherapy by Christine Wildwood
Ayurveda by Scott Gerson
Chi Kung by James MacRitchie
Chinese Medicine by Tom Williams
Colour Therapy by Pauline Wills
Flower Remedies by Christine Wildwood
Herbal Medicine by Vicki Pitman
Kinesiology by Ann Holdway
Massage by Stewart Mitchell
Reflexology by Inge Dougans with Suzanne Ellis
Shiatsu by Elaine Liechti
Skin and Body Care by Sidra Shaukat
Spiritual Healing by Jack Angelo
Vitamin Guide by Hasnain Walji

Health Essentials

ALEXANDER TECHNIQUE

Natural Poise
for Health

Richard Brennan

ELEMENT
Shaftesbury, Dorset ● Rockport, Massachusetts
Brisbane, Queensland

© Richard Brennan 1991

First published in Great Britain in 1991 by
Element Books Limited
Shaftesbury, Dorset

Published in the USA in 1991 by
Element, Inc.
42 Broadway, Rockport, MA 01966

Published in Australia in 1993 by
Element Books Limited for
Jacaranda Wiley Limited
33 Park Road, Milton, Brisbane 4064

Reprinted 1991
Reprinted 1993
Reprinted 1995

Cover design by Max Fairbrother
Cover illustration from an Eric Gill Woodcut
Illustrations by David Gifford
Typeset in Goudy by Selectmove Limited
Printed and bound in Great Britain by
Biddles Ltd, Guildford & King's Lynn

British Library Cataloguing in Publication Data
Brennan, Richard
Alexander technique.
1. Alternative therapy
I. Title II. Series
615.82

Library of Congress Cataloging in Publication
Data available

ISBN 1–85230–217–8

Note from the Publisher

Any information given in any book in the *Health Essentials* series
is not intended to be taken as a replacement for medical advice.
Any person with a condition requiring medical attention should
consult a qualified medical practitioner or suitable therapist.

This book is dedicated
to
all who are in pain

Acknowledgements

I WOULD LIKE to thank the following for their encouragement, inspiration and patience in teaching me the Alexander Technique and in the writing of this book: Cara Brennan, Tim Brennan, Evelyn Burges, Paul Collins, Margaret Farrar, David Gorman, Trish Hemmingway, Alan Mars, Camilla Mars, Clare Morris, Henry Morris, Jessica Morris, Danny Riley, Refia Sacks, Chris Stevens and many others too numerous to name.

Contents

Know Thyself

Socrates

Introduction

WHAT DO John Cleese, Roald Dahl, Aldous Huxley, Paul Newman, George Bernard Shaw, the Duchess of York and Sting all have in common? 'Not a lot' is maybe your first thought, and yet they have all spoken of the great benefits that they have received from practising the Alexander Technique.

But why do people of such varied backgrounds and lifestyles all praise the Technique so highly? What are the benefits that they have gained? I will endeavour to answer these questions at a later stage.

Many people today have heard of the Alexander Technique and more and more articles in magazines and newspapers discuss it. 'But what is the Alexander Technique exactly?' I hear many people say. There seems to be an air of mystery surrounding it and this is the very reason why I have written this book. I hope to present the Technique in such a way that it can be understood by anyone, because I feel that it is everyone's right as a human being to understand themselves more fully. The Alexander Technique has far-reaching consequences in our lives, not only on a physical level; it can greatly change our mental and emotional outlook on life.

Some readers may quickly get a sense of what is being talked about, others may take longer. So may I suggest that you read through the book and then study each chapter in turn until you feel that you have grasped the concepts.

1

What is the Alexander Technique?

All inquiry and learning is but recollection.

Socrates

THE ALEXANDER TECHNIQUE is often viewed as a technique of breathing and posture, but this is only a small part of what it really involves. It is, in truth, a method of becoming more aware of ourselves as we go about our everyday activities. We soon begin to notice, when performing the simplest of tasks, that we may be putting an enormous strain on our bodies without realizing it.

With the help of a teacher the Alexander Technique enables us to let go of many tensions that may have gone unnoticed for months or even years. These tensions are often responsible for aches and pains that accumulate with age. As any doctor will tell you, stress can be the root cause of both physical and mental disease, yet we do little to find out how these tensions first come about.

Simply sitting or standing in an unbalanced way will cause certain muscles to be constantly under stress. If these ways of standing and sitting become habitual then, sooner or later, we will have to pay the price and sometimes it is a very expensive one indeed. One of the most common consequences, here in England, is backache, with many millions of sufferers incapacitated every week. Other effects of bad posture and mal-coordination are high blood pressure, migraine, asthma, arthritis, depression and insomnia, to name but a few.

Many of our modern methods of dealing with such problems

revolve around the use of powerful drugs to suppress the painful symptoms; these drugs often have unfavourable side effects. We very rarely find out the reason why we have the ailments in the first place. The Alexander Technique does just this; by putting into practice the principles of the Technique we are able to move in a balanced and coordinated way so that tensions are not retained in our bodies.

It is easy to see the natural grace of young children as they play on the beach or in the park; but we slowly start to lose this agility of movement as the pressures of life mould us into our clumsy adult form. By the age of nine or ten the process is often under way, to the extent that I have often treated children as young as ten or eleven for backaches and headaches.

By moving in a different way we can soon regain an ease of movement that had been forgotten; many people report feeling lighter and freer after a course of lessons in the Technique. How we physically feel will, of course, affect our mental and emotional states, and I often find that people become less irritable and much more at ease with themselves. This can have a rippling effect on those close by, and family and friends alike have remarked on the improved temperament of people who begin to practise the Alexander Technique.

An Alexander Technique lesson consists of two parts:

1. To help the pupil detect and let go of excessive tension that has been held unconsciously in the body.
2. To help the pupil find different ways of moving that are easier and more efficient, thus reducing wear and tear on body structure and internal organs.

In the first instance you may be asked to lie face up on a table; there will be no need to remove your clothes apart from your shoes. The teacher will then ask you neither to resist nor help while he gently moves your head and limbs. It never hurts, as is sometimes the case in physiotherapy or other therapies, since the movements are often very small. When the teacher finds some resistance due to muscular tension he will then ask you to relax the limb that you have been tensing; he may suggest ways to help you to do this. At the end of a half-hour session, the difference in how you feel may well be quite dramatic. You will feel much lighter, as gravity will be working on you in a very different way. Sometimes, long-standing aches and pains are known to disappear completely, much to the pupil's amazement.

The teacher will then take you through a series of movements so that he will be able to find out when you are tensing your muscles unnecessarily. You will explore new ways of moving to bring about a more natural coordination of the body. This will produce a greater sense of well-being and you will have more energy left to do the things you want to, instead of collapsing in front of the television. Have you ever wondered where children get all their energy from? Their actions are much more efficient than ours and therefore they still have lots of energy left when we feel exhausted.

The Alexander Technique is referred to as a re-education rather than a therapy, because the practitioner is teaching you about yourself. If any disease is cured in the process then it will be you that is curing yourself.

Although the effects of the Technique can be far reaching it is, at the same time, simple and can be easily understood by everyone. The important qualities to have are patience and a willingness to learn about oneself. In some cases people cannot grasp some of the basic principles because they are looking for something more complicated.

The Alexander Technique is often grouped with various forms of complementary medicines, but it stands in its own right, being quite unique. This is because it gives each and every one of us the responsibility for our own well-being. We are encouraged to think for ourselves, so it is a useful tool for awareness and self-development – about which the world is becoming more interested.

When we begin to apply the principles in our lives we see that we are not learning anything new; rather, we are unlearning. Alexander was often heard to say, 'If you stop doing the wrong thing the right thing will happen

4

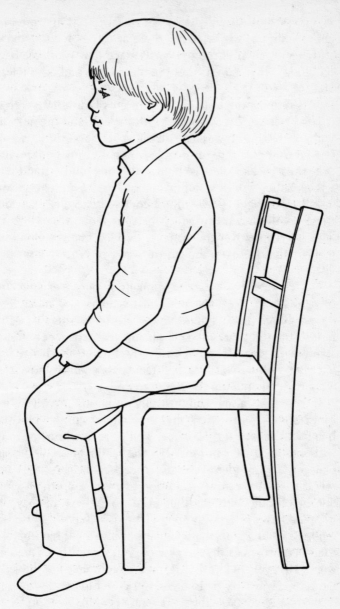

Fig. 1. *Children naturally sit in an upright manner*

automatically'. It really does not matter what age you are (I am teaching a lady of eighty-three at the moment), you can still regain much of the poise and grace that you once had in childhood. If you do not believe me, just go and have a lesson and see for yourself.

It is astonishing how many of us grossly interfere with the natural workings of our bodies. Just look around the next time you are waiting in a queue at the supermarket or the bank, and you are bound to see people who have hunched shoulders or arched backs. Many of them will not even be standing up straight; they will be standing on one leg or leaning backwards at quite an angle. They will, of course, be totally unaware of these bodily distortions which become more acute with age. This is because over the years we develop many habits which feel comfortable even though they may be putting a strain on us.

We very rarely give much thought to ourselves apart from how we look. We may spend many hours and hundreds of pounds improving our appearance yet, to me, there is nothing more attractive than someone who moves with grace and sits or stands with poise. The Alexander Technique also has the side effect of making you look and feel years younger, something we spend much of our life trying to do.

If you play a musical instrument or are involved in a sport of any kind then the Technique will be especially helpful as it will increase your ability to perform for longer without the usual tensions. All the major music and drama colleges have resident Alexander teachers because they have found that many students are forced to give up their careers due to chronic tensions that arise from the way they hold their bodies while performing. Not only have the students reported feeling much better, but they also say it has improved their performances. In the case of professional sportsmen and women in every field, the Alexander Technique has proved all important when trying to break world records.

So, as you can see, there are many benefits in applying the Technique in your life. You may wish to use it as a prevention against future ill-health, a less expensive insurance than any of the insurance policies on the market today. It is widely agreed that prevention is better than cure, but how many people really take steps in order to ensure good health later in life? I am naturally biased, being a teacher of the Alexander Technique, but I cannot help thinking that if some of the basic principles were taught in our schools then millions of people would not suffer so greatly later on in life. This would save our National Health Service many millions of pounds each year, as well as preventing the great loss to our industries because of countless working days wasted due to ill-health.

Being aware of one's body is nothing new. People involved with the martial arts have realized the importance for many thousands of years. They knew that the mind can have a marked effect upon how one moves, and the same ideas are still used today.

A THERAPY OR AN EDUCATION?

Many people think that the Alexander Technique is another therapy similar to homoeopathy, osteopathy and acupuncture. It is very different, however, because it involves the pupil consciously letting go of unnecessary tension. The effects of Alexander's work may be, and very often are, therapeutic, but it is much more a process by which pupils learn how they can help themselves. So the pupil is taking an active part in the process and the teacher cannot do anything without his or her willingness.

If we can find the reason for our aches or pains then it does not take long to put things right. Alexander once said, 'You can change the habits of a lifetime in a few moments, if you just use your brains.' I personally have been a witness to this time and time again, and have been very surprised at how quickly so many people have changed.

Many of our common actions, like sitting, standing or walking, have to be learned anew and these new movements may, at first, feel very strange. The habitual way in which we move may be the very cause of many tensions which so often lead to sickness and pain, but to us that way of living has become a part of us.

These tensions in our bodies begin to result in pain which, of course, makes us more tense, and so a vicious cycle is set up. If we can start to learn how to use our bodies in a different way then the muscular tensions will slowly disappear. These different ways of moving are not new to us, they are the ways we moved as children – but because of internal and external pressures we have forgotten them. I myself would therefore call the Alexander Technique a method of re-education, a way of re-discovering the natural grace of movement which is inherent in each and every one of us.

If you do decide to have a course of lessons then it is important to realize that this re-education does take time and often it is hard to understand what is happening for the first six or seven lessons. Eventually, however, you will have learned a technique which you can use to help yourself for the rest of your life. In one of my evening classes I met a lady who had had lessons from Alexander himself more than fifty years ago; she claimed that it had been the main reason why she had been so fit and free from illness throughout her life. She was nearly eighty and the last time I heard from her she was off to France to do some serious walking in the Alps.

There is nothing like pain to motivate people into looking at themselves, but if people do come for lessons, before the tensions or pain are too bad, then often they may not need so many lessons. The main qualities to have in this process are an open mind and a willingness to look at oneself.

MIND, BODY AND SPIRIT UNITY

Alexander was convinced that the mind, body and spirit were interconnected. In other words, the way we think can affect

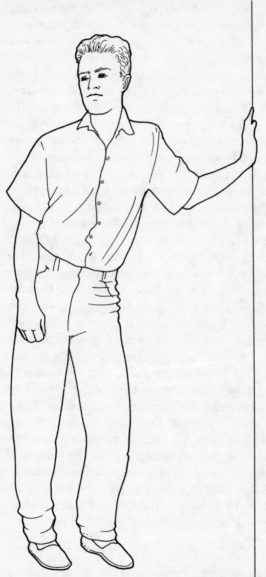

Fig. 2. A common standing position – the whole body alignment is distorted causing excess muscular tension

the way we feel and can often be at the bottom of many tensions or diseases. Similarly, the way in which we sit or stand can alter the way in which we feel or think.

This can easily be seen in a patient suffering from depression– they will invariably be sitting in a slumped manner with rounded shoulders and a collapsed chest. This will interfere with their breathing and, ultimately, with the body's life energy. Whenever movement is to take place there has to be an enormous amount of effort to bring a person out of his slumped posture, so most of the time he cannot be bothered to perform even simple tasks. This will only add to his reasons for being depressed, and so a vicious cycle is set up.

The way in which we think is as much a part of the Alexander Technique as the way in which we move. In essence the Technique is a way of using our minds in a conscious manner so that we are able efficiently to direct our bodies in order to keep them as stress-free as possible. This, in turn, will allow the natural healing processes to function as effectively as possible.

Tension that is allowed to build up unnoticed will interfere with the circulatory, respiratory and nervous systems. This will eventually lead to many of the illnesses that we see today, most of which could be avoided altogether. These tensions are merely a reflection of the stressed condition of our minds. We are trained from an early age to be goal-orientated or, as Alexander described it, 'end-gaining'. Most of us spend very little time just 'being', we are always doing this or that in our very busy schedules. But are we human beings or human doers? Due to our modern civilization I fear that we are becoming the latter. How many of us stop just for a moment and ask ourselves, 'Am I doing what I really want to do with my life or am I finding that I have little or no choice in the matter?'

The Alexander Technique is about having free choice on every level, without which we are only surviving and not living. We seem to be living in a rat-race, yet it is important

10

to remember that it does not matter who wins, that person is still a rat.

Alexander named his first book, *Man's Supreme Inheritance*. He believed that consciousness was man's birthright and the next stage in our evolutionary development, yet most of the time we are ruled by time and fear. We spend most of our time performing actions for others, rather than because it is what we really want to do. He once said, 'Everyone wants to change and yet remain the same'. It reminds me of the joke, 'How many psychotherapists does it take to change a light bulb?' The answer is 'one, but the light bulb has got to want to change'.

So we have to be prepared to change our way of thinking if we are ever to free our bodies from stresses and strains. The benefits are enormous. We have so much to gain and so little to lose; a willingness to learn about ourselves is the only essential requirement. Once we are able to let go of the tensions that imprison both mind and body, then we will begin to experience the joy of life that we once had as children.

AWARENESS

The first step to take when learning the Alexander Technique is to try to become more aware of yourself, how you go about your activities as well as what you are thinking as you do them. This is quite hard at first, but gets easier with practice. Later on in this book you will find exercises that will help awareness in even the simplest of actions.

You may discover that a comfortable habit of standing or sitting is very stressful. Have you ever caught sight of yourself in a shop window or on a video, and got a shock because you did not know that you moved like that? It is often such an experience that motivates the starting of Alexander lessons because a person sees that if he or she carries on in the same way there will be serious problems later on in life.

Pain is the other main reason why many people are forced to look at themselves, yet the signs of tension have been present for many years. Most of us are too busy with our lives to even notice tension and we are often taken by surprise when our body starts to fail. If we learn to become more aware of ourselves then we may well be able to avoid many ailments later on in life.

Most of the time we are thinking about anything but the task at hand; we are rarely in the present moment. The Alexander Technique is a very practical method which enables us to be conscious of each moment; this enhances the quality of our life and enables us to live life to the full.

TIME

If there is one factor most responsible for tension, it is time. Our civilization is ruled by it. From the age of five when we first start school, we are under a pressure to be at certain places at certain times. It is so obvious, standing outside the school gates at nine o'clock every day, that getting their children ready on time has caused mothers a great deal of stress and anxiety. As children, we live in another world, as do people in less developed countries. This world is ruled by the five senses. A child will naturally be drawn to attractive things that he sees or hears. But as adults we usually have a preconceived plan of what our day is going to be like and, if we get behind in our schedule, then we tend to become tense. When I started having Alexander lessons I noticed that when I was late for an appointment, which was quite often, I started to tense my neck muscles and poke my head forward as though this would get me there sooner. That neck tension had always been there in those circumstances, but I had not noticed it. This tension remained in my body even when I had reached my destination and eventually caused headaches, neck problems and a general lack of coordination. I often remember this very thought-provoking saying: Man says that

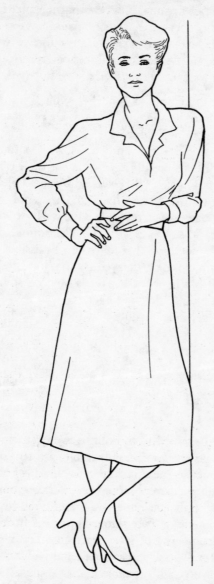

Fig. 3. *The way in which we stand can put many muscles under stress without us noticing*

13

time is passing away, but time says that it is man that passes away.

Most people will argue that we have to live within these time structures unless we drop out of society; this is true, but there is much we can do to alleviate stress:

1. Leave plenty of time to get where you are going. This is especially important when hold-ups are possible, such as in heavy traffic or at road-works.
2. Try not to undertake too much. Most of us find it hard to say no to friends or colleagues and we then take on more than we can manage; this causes an incredible amount of tension as we rush around trying to get all our jobs finished before the deadlines which we have set for ourselves. It is a good idea to say, 'Yes – if I have the time,' rather than commit to something that may not be possible.
3. If you are unavoidably delayed try to phone and let people know what has happened. This is obvious advice but it is often the obvious that we forget.
4. If you are behind schedule and there is nothing you can do about it – RELAX. This is easier said than done, but it is very important that you try. It is easy to see tense and irritated drivers who are late for work, and this can so easily lead to accidents. It is always when we are rushing that we knock the milk over or forget to turn off the iron, which causes us to be later still.

Tensions stay in our body without us even realizing, but they only manifest years later as, for example, arthritis or migraine. In order to practise the Alexander Technique you will need to give yourself time to observe how you use your body, but this does not mean you have to do things slowly. Just give yourself a moment or two before acting to find the easiest and most efficient way of going about it. You nearly always save yourself time. Look at a cat, for example: it always pauses before it jumps up onto the table in order to assimilate all the information needed to carry out the action; yet the cat is one of the fastest creatures on Earth.

Alexander called this process of stopping and thinking about actions before carrying them out – INHIBITION. This should not be confused with the Freudian term which means suppression of feeling. In Chapter 4 we will look at this process of inhibition in detail.

FEAR

Fear is the other main factor which can cause tension within our bodies:

Fear of Falling

As children we are always falling over and we never really seem to hurt ourselves yet, as we get older, one fall can put us out of action for months. Why is this? As we get older our muscles grow more and more tense; when we fall, the fear causes even more muscular tension and we hit the ground as a rigid structure, which is highly vulnerable to breakage and fracture. An interesting fact is that most hip operations, as a result of falling, are caused by muscle tension breaking the hip before the person has even reached the ground. A frightening thought, but a good example of how stressed muscles can become. The reason why people who faint do not hurt themselves is because their muscles are relaxed as they are unable consciously to tense. The same applies to people who fall over when they are drunk.

Fear of Criticism

One can easily see the muscle tension that is present when children are being reprimanded; if this happens often enough at school or at home then these tensions can easily become fixed in their bodies.

The list of fears is a long one, from the fear of losing one's job to the fear of death, and each one will cause stress within our bodies without us even realizing it. It is often the case that we are completely unaware of many of the fears from which we suffer.

The Alexander Technique can help to release much of this muscular tension before it is able to do real, or even irreversible, damage. We only have this one body, so the way in which we use it is of the utmost importance. It is often the case that we look after our house or our car better than we look after ourselves, but both our house and our car can be replaced – our bodies cannot.

2

The History of the Alexander Technique

The cure of the part should not be attempted without treatment of the whole.

Plato

HOW IT ALL BEGAN

FREDERICK MATTHIAS ALEXANDER, the progenitor of the Alexander Technique, was born in Australia on 20 January 1869. He was the eldest child of John and Betsy Alexander who lived in Wynyard, a small town on the north-west coast of Tasmania. John was a farmer and Betsy was the local nurse and midwife. Frederick (or F.M. as his friends used to call him) was born prematurely and was not expected to live more than a few weeks; it was only due to his mother's great love for her child that he did survive.

Frederick was plagued with one illness after another throughout his childhood, mainly suffering from asthma and other breathing problems. As a result, he had to be taken away from school and was given private tuition in the evenings from the local school teacher. This left plenty of free time during the day which he spent with his father's horses; he gradually became an expert at training and managing them. At this time he acquired his sensitivity of touch which proved to be invaluable later in his career.

At the age of eleven his health slowly began to improve; by the time he was seventeen financial hardship within the family forced Frederick to leave the outdoor life that he had grown to love so much. He began employment in the office of a tin-mining company at the nearby town of Mount Bischoff. In his spare time he became more and more interested in amateur dramatics, as well as teaching himself to play the violin.

After three years he had saved up enough money to travel to Melbourne where he stayed with his uncle. During the next three months Alexander spent all his hard-earned money visiting the theatre, art galleries or going to concerts. He had decided to train to be a reciter.

He then took various jobs including that of a clerk to an estate agent, a shop assistant in a department store and even as a tea taster for a firm of tea merchants. This paid for his training which he did in the evenings and at weekends. Alexander very quickly established an excellent reputation as an actor and reciter and soon formed his own theatre company which specialized in one-man Shakespearean recitals. He was particularly fond of *The Merchant of Venice* and *Hamlet*.

All went well for a short while, but then his childhood respiratory problems returned. His voice became hoarse and the audience began to notice that he was sucking in air loudly between sentences. On one occasion Alexander completely lost his voice during one of his performances. This was a great blow to his confidence and he became reluctant to accept engagements for fear of losing his voice at a crucial moment in front of an audience. Not only was his career in jeopardy, but also the theatre that he had grown to love and treasure so much. He became desperate and was willing to try anything in search for a solution to his problem. Alexander sought the advice of numerous doctors and voice trainers who gave him different medicines or voice exercises, but this only brought him temporary relief.

Finally, one of the doctors who had been advising him prescribed complete rest of the voice for a full two weeks before his next recital. The doctor assured Alexander that, if he followed these instructions exactly, his voice would return to normal. Alexander, being a very determined man, went the next two weeks hardly uttering a word. At the beginning of his next performance his voice was crystal clear, being completely free from the previous defects. His spirits lifted only to be dashed half an hour later when the hoarseness reappeared. By the end of the evening he described his voice as being in the most distressing condition, the problem had returned so acutely that he was hardly able to speak.

Alexander's disappointment was indescribable; he now thought that he would never again be able to have more than temporary relief. He believed that he would have to give up a career to which he was deeply committed and which had promised to be highly successful.

The very next day he went back to the doctor to tell him what had happened. The doctor then told Alexander that he must go on with the treatment. Alexander could see no point at all in doing this and flatly refused. If his voice had been alright at the beginning of his performance, and yet he could hardly speak by the end, then it must be a result of something that he was doing while reciting that was causing the problem. The doctor thought for a moment and then nodded in agreement. Alexander asked if the doctor knew what that something was, but he could not give him any answer.

So Alexander left the surgery determined that he, himself, was going to find out the solution to his curious problem. He did exactly that, little knowing that he was about to stumble upon one of the greatest discoveries of this century.

It is important to remember that it was Alexander's all-consuming passion for the theatre that gave him the determination to find out the cause of his hoarseness. He was faced with one setback after another, as we shall see, and most people would have given up along the way. It took him seven long and difficult years to find out where he was going wrong.

The story that follows can be likened to a tale of exploration, not a new land that he stumbled across, but an important discovery, not only for himself but for the whole of mankind.

FIRST DISCOVERIES

After Alexander's conversation with his doctor he was left with only two leads; these were as follows:

1. When he rested his voice, or only spoke normally, then the hoarseness disappeared.
2. When he began to project his voice during recitals then the hoarseness always returned.

He began to experiment on himself. He started to speak and then to recite in front of a mirror. After a short while Alexander noticed that he was doing three things while reciting; these actions were not present when using his normal speaking voice:

1. He tended to pull his head back and down onto his spine with an enormous amount of tension.
2. He depressed his larynx, the site of the vocal cords.
3. He began to suck in air through his mouth, producing a gasping sound.

After many months of careful observation he realized that he was doing exactly the same thing while talking, but to a much lesser extent, and that was why his speaking habits had gone undetected. He had been using a great deal of unnecessary and inappropriate tension when reciting. This tension was, indeed, the root cause of his problem.

When Alexander came to correct his problem, however, he began to experience great difficulties. While still using the mirror he tried not to tense his neck muscles, nor to depress his larynx, nor to make the gasping sounds. He found that he was unable to do anything to improve the condition of his larynx or his breathing, but he was able to stop pulling his head back. This indicated to him that the tension in his neck was causing the other two problems.

At this point he wrote in his journal,

The importance of this discovery cannot be over-estimated, for through it I was led on to the further discovery of the Primary Control of the workings of all the mechanisms of the human organisms, and this marked the first important stage of my investigation.

The Primary Control

What did Alexander mean by the Primary Control, a phrase that will recur throughout this book?

The Primary Control acts as the main reflex in the body. It is situated in the area of the neck and governs all the other reflexes of our body. Because of this our extremely complex mechanisms become comparatively simple to organize. As it is the relationship of the head to the rest of the body; it is often referred to as 'the head, neck, back relationship'.

It is essential to point out that the Primary Control relationship is not one of position, but one of freedom. When this relationship is interfered with, due to excessive muscular tension, it can offset all the other reflexes throughout the body. This, in turn, will cause a lack of coordination and balance which will lead to inefficiency of movement. A good example of this can be seen in riding. When a rider wishes to stop a horse he, or she, pulls the horse's head back by use of the reins. The animal immediately loses its coordination and soon comes to a standstill.

It is also worth noting that, due to the fact that people have a lack of certain sense receptors in the neck, it is very difficult to tell when you are tensing your neck muscles and when you are not.

TENSION LEADS TO MORE TENSION

After his initial discovery of the Primary Control, Alexander also noticed that when he was able to prevent tension from building up in his neck muscles, then the hoarseness in his voice decreased accordingly. When he was later examined by several doctors, a considerable improvement of his throat and vocal cords had taken place. This showed that the way he used himself when reciting had a marked effect on his voice and breathing.

The implications of this observation were very far-reaching and, as the months passed, Alexander slowly began to notice that, when he pulled his head back, he also had a tendency to lift his chest and shorten his whole stature. Fascinated with his new discovery he went on experimenting and then found he was also arching and narrowing his back.

This observation led him to his third important realization, namely, that the tension that he had seen in his neck was causing other tensions throughout his whole structure.

FAULTY SENSORY PERCEPTION

Alexander started to examine the effects that shortening and lengthening of his body had on his voice. He discovered that the hoarseness came back only when he pulled his head back and down onto his spine and so shortened his stature with excessive tension. At this discovery he felt as though he was really achieving something. Not only had he spotted excessive muscular tension throughout his body, but now he thought he knew how to correct it. All he had to do was to put his head forward and up, instead of pulling it back and down, and his problem would be solved.

It was not as easy as that because, when he put his head forward, he saw in the mirror that he was still lifting his chest and arching his back. He could hardly believe his eyes. At this point he was overcome with bitter disappointment. He nearly gave up, not knowing what to do next.

Alexander then placed two extra mirrors either side of the original mirror that he had been using. He quickly noticed that, although he had been convinced that he was putting his head forward, he was in fact pulling his head back with even more tension than before.

He realized that he was a victim of faulty sensory perception. This simply means that he felt that he was doing one thing when, in fact, he was really doing the opposite. It was only later that he found out that nearly everyone suffers from the same delusion in one form or another; at the time he was convinced that it was his own personal idiosyncrasy. There was nothing for it but to persevere. He continued for several months experimenting with both successes and failures. As he did, he began to notice more tensions in his legs, feet and even his toes. His toes were contracted and bent downward so that his feet were very arched. This threw his weight onto the outside of the feet which affected his whole balance, causing excessive stress throughout his entire body.

Slowly it dawned on Alexander that the tension that he had first noticed was not of specific parts, as he had first presumed, but of himself as a whole being. He was still convinced that if he could somehow get rid of the tension in the neck then the other problems would automatically be resolved. He stopped all experimentation at this stage to examine the information he had gathered so far. The important issues that he noted were these:

1. The fact that he was pulling his head back and down, when he thought he was putting it forward and up, was positive proof that he could no longer trust his physical impressions.
2. These untrustworthy impressions were both unconscious and instinctive.
3. This faulty sensory perception, as he called it, was an inseparable part of an habitual use of himself.
4. This habit was a direct result of an instinctive response to the stimulus of reciting.

In short, he had developed a habit of increasing muscular tension whenever he started reciting. Alexander had, up to now, been completely ignorant of this habit, and anything that he did to change it only made the situation worse. It dawned on him that, if he was ever able to cure the persistent

23

hoarseness in his voice, he must first replace his old instinctive habits with a new and conscious use of himself.

DIRECTIONS

Alexander started to direct his actions by inventing orders which he gave to himself when standing, sitting and reciting. He called these orders 'directions'. The main three were:

1. Allow the neck to be free.
2. Allow the head to go forward and upward.
3. Allow the back to lengthen and widen.

These directions were in complete contradiction to his old habits and Alexander found they were successful in bringing about the change that he had sought for so long.

He did have one last setback, however: as long as he was not reciting he was free from tension in the neck but, as soon as he began to use his voice, all his old habits returned. It seemed to him that he had come so far in discovering so much about his problem but was unable to bring about any substantial change.

INHIBITION

In exasperation he gave up trying to 'do' anything to reach his goal. To his amazement, the very results that he had been after for several years were achieved. At last he saw that, if he was ever to eliminate his old habits, then he must refuse to do anything at all until he had given himself the directions. Alexander called this process 'inhibition'.

As previously mentioned, this is not the type of inhibition talked of in Freudian books which, in that context, means to suppress feelings. Inhibition, as recommended by Alexander, is the ability to pause for a moment until we are adequately prepared to carry out actions satisfactorily. A good example of this is a cat. A cat inhibits the desire to chase the bird until it is ready so that it has the highest chance of success.

So Alexander worked out a technique that not only freed him from the tendency which was at the bottom of his vocal troubles, but also cured his asthma from which he had suffered from birth.

TEACHING OTHERS

He returned to his much loved reciting career. By this time there was a great interest in how he had overcome his problem when so many other treatments had failed. Soon Alexander found himself teaching fellow actors, with similar problems, what he had learned.

Before long many people from far and wide had heard about his successes, and doctors and specialists began to send him some of their patients. Within a few months he was teaching full-time.

As his workload increased he asked his brother, Albert Redden Alexander (nick-named A.R. for short) to join him. Fredrick taught his brother his technique in a short time and the two brothers worked side by side, often having long discussions about the technique, modifying it as they went along.

In 1903 J.W. Stewart McKay, a prominent surgeon in Sydney, persuaded Alexander to go to London so that he could bring his valuable technique before the world. So in the spring of 1904 he left his homeland, never to return.

He arrived in London some months later with letters of introduction to both actors and physicians. He was soon joined by his brother and the two of them set up a practice in the Army and Navy Mansions on Victoria Street. As in Australia, they were soon working flat out with people coming to them from all walks of life. Many of the leading actors of that day came to him and some of them, such as Sir Henry Irving, used to have his professional help between acts of their plays.

Between 1906 and 1908 Alexander published pamphlets and articles, both privately and in the press, and in 1910 his first book, entitled *Man's Supreme Inheritance*, was published. At the beginning of the First World War he sailed for the United States of America and spent the next ten years dividing his teaching between there and England. He continued to write, publishing a further two books entitled *Conscious Control* and *Constructive Conscious Control*.

In 1920 Alexander married the actress Edith Page, a fellow Australian, but his marriage was not particularly happy and for the most part they lived apart. She was not in favour of the work which he so loved, yet he always treated her with affection. After a couple of years they adopted a child which they named Peggy, of whom he was very fond.

In the mid 1920s a class was set up in London; in 1934 this became a school at Penhill in Kent. His Technique became fundamental to the whole school curriculum. Alexander appreciated that since most problems start in early life it should be possible to avoid these with the right teaching. By learning his Technique children became more upright and showed greater enquiry, both physically and mentally. He was well pleased with the fruits that his Technique bore at the school.

When Alexander reached the age of sixty he was persuaded by many friends, afraid that his most valuable secrets would die with him, to set up a training school to teach others to be teachers of his technique. So, in 1931, he began to train teachers to carry on his work; this school was set up in his home at 16 Ashley Place in London SW1 and it continued up to his death in October 1955.

Throughout his life Alexander tried to get his work recognized by the medical profession, but to little avail. It is true that the *British Medical Journal* wrote favourably about his technique in 1930: 'Mr. Alexander's work is of first class importance and investigation by the medical profession is imperative.' Again, in 1937, nineteen doctors published a letter in the *BMJ* stating that they were satisfied, through

26

personal experience, that Alexander's teaching was very beneficial in the cure and prevention of many diseases. They called upon their profession to investigate his claims and to include the Alexander Technique in the medical curriculum of trainee doctors. Unfortunately, for many millions of people, no action was taken on either occasion.

Even the Nobel prize winners Nikolaas Tinbergen and Sir Charles Sherrington spoke of Alexander's work with very high regard; Nikolaas Tinbergen even dedicated his prize-winning speech to Alexander, but even to this day Alexander has not really received the recognition he so richly deserves. Among his many pupils were the authors George Bernard Shaw and Aldous Huxley, the scientists Professor Raymond Dart, Professor George E. Coghill and Professor Frank Pierce Jones, as well as many well-known actors – too numerous to list in full.

Today there are thousands of trained teachers throughout the world carrying on his work nearly forty years after his death. The numbers are growing as the demand ever increases.

3

What Can the Technique Do for You?

Every man, woman and child holds the possibility of physical perfection; it rests with each one of us to attain it by personal understanding and effort.

Frederick Matthias Alexander

Y OU MAY BE one of those millions of people suffering from backache, stiff neck, headaches, arthritis or other symptoms for which there seems to be no answer. The Alexander Technique does not set out to cure specific symptoms, but it does help to uncover and change those harmful and unconscious habit patterns which, all too often, are the underlying cause of a problem.

You may be suffering from stress as a result of work or other numerous circumstances. The Technique will help you to look more closely at your reactions in everyday situations and will enable you to see clearly for yourself how, without realizing it, you contribute to the build-up of excessive tension in your life. When you are made aware of this you can consciously choose not to react in a stressed way and you will therefore be able to maintain a calmness even when life becomes hectic.

Or you might be a musician, an actor, a dancer, a singer or a sports person who relies on functioning to peak efficiency in order to obtain the best results. The Alexander Technique, by giving a means to release the excessive build-up of tension, helps you to perform much nearer to your maximum ability with the minimum amount of effort.

Lastly, you may be perfectly healthy but are one of those

increasing number of people who want to take responsibility for their own well-being and wish to discover more about themselves. You can use the Alexander Technique as a preventative measure: after all, prevention is better than cure.

These are only a few of the more common applications of the Technique. It can be used by anyone to improve whatever it is that interests him or her. The only requirements are patience, a willingness to learn and a readiness to let go of the habits of a lifetime.

HABITS

We all have habits that we aware of, but the habits that Alexander referred to are below our level of consciousness. In other words, we are completely unaware of them, usually because our mind is somewhere else.

At any given moment our mind is wandering into the future or into the past; we are very rarely present in the here and now. Alexander often referred to this condition as the 'mind-wandering habit' which will often lead us to use our bodies in a very uncoordinated way, without even realizing it. Have you ever been walking or driving towards a destination and completely missed your turning because your mind was somewhere else? I am sure the answer is yes; we all do it from time to time. Every day, we are preoccupied with thoughts without even noticing it. While this is happening we may get into standing, walking or sitting in ways that are a strain on the body. If we do this often enough, and most of us do, then these ways of being become habitual and eventually the muscle tension that is required for these unnatural positions becomes fixed into our body. Very soon this rigidity starts to restrict movements and by the time we reach old age we can barely get around. Much of this stiffness is avoidable if we act early enough and, through having Alexander lessons, much of the stiffness can be erased from our lives. It is important to remember that it is never too late and no one is beyond help.

It is necessary to understand that the tightness in one set of muscles will invariably affect our whole body balance. After correcting the posture we will find that movements become easier and we will sense a lightness that has not been present since childhood. We begin to perform activities with greater efficiency and therefore have much more energy at the end of the day.

The same effects may be achieved by having a massage but, unlike a massage, the feeling of lightness can last for days and we can eventually learn how to release tension for ourselves.

Since the very basis of the Technique rests upon Alexander's discovery that it was impossible to separate the physical, emotional and mental states from each other, then it follows that the way in which we use our bodies will, in turn, alter the way in which we think and how we feel emotionally. Unhappiness and feelings of unfulfillment, therefore, must stem from the way in which we move in this world. By practising the Alexander Technique feelings and thoughts can alter. Alexander wrote on the subject of unhappiness:

I shall now endeavour to show that the lack of real happiness manifested by the majority of adults today is due to the fact that they are experiencing, not an improving, but a continually deteriorating use of their psycho-physical selves. This is associated with those defects, imperfections, undesirable traits of character, disposition, temperament, etc., characteristic of imperfectly coordinated people struggling through life beset with certain maladjustments of the psycho-physical organism, which are actually setting up conditions of irritation and pressure during both sleeping and waking hours. Whilst the maladjustments remain present, these malconditions increase day by day and week by week, and foster that unsatisfactory state which we call 'Unhappiness'.

In short, the habitual way of being that so many of us are encouraged to fall into from a very early age is bound to affect our physical, mental and even our spiritual well-being. This will encourage undesirable qualities such as frustration, anger, lack of confidence and a general feeling of dissatisfaction with life in general. These states will, in turn, begin to become habitual.

Not one of us begins life feeling angry or frustrated, no one as an infant is dissatisfied or lacks feelings of self-worth. These are states that we acquire as life's internal and external pressures take their toll. Just take a careful look the next time you are out shopping; how many people look happy?

Every experience that we have is transmitted into muscular tension. The trouble is that we forget to let go of the tension. Animals also have tensions when they are in activity, but they instinctively know how to relax.

So the Alexander Technique not only helps posture and coordination, it also balances emotions and helps to bring us peace of mind.

Later on in this chapter you will see how it has helped specific people in their lives, but first I would like to show how the technique can help some of the more common ailments that many people suffer today.

Backache

An estimated million people are off work with back pain each week in England alone. This figure does not include school children, students, housewives, mothers with small children, senior citizens, or people who are unemployed; nor does it include those many people who struggle into work with an aching back. The cost to industry is over £250,000,000 each year, to say nothing of the individual's suffering or loss of income. Much of this is completely avoidable. By having Alexander lessons an individual would be able to learn how to sit, stand or pick objects up so that they do not put so much strain on the back muscles, thus bringing instant relief to their back.

Stiff Neck or Frozen Shoulders

This again is entirely due to excess muscle tension and, with the help of a teacher, the pupil can learn to let go of the muscles that are causing the problem.

Hypertension

This again is a very common problem and is more usually known as high blood pressure. Many of the arteries and veins of the circulation system run through the muscles of the body. If these muscles are in a constant state of tension, then they become hardened; this restricts the flow of blood to and from the heart. The heart has then got to work harder and harder to keep the flow of blood going, thus causing high blood pressure.

Chris Stevens, a physicist and Alexander teacher, has performed experiments on people suffering from hypertension and has shown that Alexander lessons lower blood pressure significantly.

Headaches and Migraine

While working on people who suffer from these conditions I have always found that the neck muscles are extremely tight. With headaches the pain will almost always disappear (while I am working on them) as soon as they release the tension that has caused the pain. With migraines results often take longer, but the attacks soon become less frequent and their intensity decreases.

Asthma

As you will remember from Chapter 2 Alexander himself suffered from asthma very badly as a child. After developing his technique he was free from all his respiratory problems and they never bothered him again throughout his life.

Arthritis

Arthritis is yet another very common illness in today's society. It is most common in older people and it is often believed that there is no cure because it is a sign that the body is wearing out. Most people are just given pain-killers to cope with the condition. What is happening is that two bones in the body are being pulled together and are wearing each other out. Very few of us stop to ask what it is that is pulling them together. The muscles that connect the two bones are clearly under a colossal amount of tension and this is pulling these two bones together. Once the pressure is reduced then the bones can heal themselves because bone is, like everything in the body, a living tissue.

Depression

Normally, depression can only be treated with powerful drugs which have many side effects. My father, a doctor, suffered from depression throughout his life. He could only get temporary relief from certain drugs and it was believed that the same drug contributed to the hardening of the liver which led to his death. I wish to point out that, of course, drugs do have their place and many people gain tremendous relief from them, but they are not in most cases the long-term solution to so many of our problems. In the case of depression, it is easy to see the body shape which accompanies such a condition. If you can alter the shape through muscle release then the mental and emotional condition of the person will also change.

Breathing and Voice

Treatment for breathing difficulties requires a relaxation of certain muscles to free the rib-cage; then the breathing will automatically start working naturally. As Alexander was often heard to say – if you stop doing the wrong thing, then the right thing will emerge naturally.

There are so many diseases that can be helped by the Alexander Technique because, whatever problem we may have, the remedy is always the same: find out what it is that is causing the problem, stop doing whatever it is and then you will soon start to feel better. This is a very simple philosophy but, in my experience, I have seen it work time and time again. I myself have often been surprised at how quickly so many people feel the benefit.

The best way to understand how people, from all walks of life, can be helped is to hear from them personally, so I asked several people from my classes in Devon to write a short summary about how the Alexander Technique had helped them. I have not changed in any way the words in which they expressed themselves.

CASE HISTORIES

One great feature of Mr. Alexander's system as seen in practical use is that the individual loses every suggestion of strain. He becomes perfectly 'lissom' in body; all strains and tensions disappear, and his body works like an oiled machine. Moreover, his system has a reflex result upon the mind of the patient, and a general condition of buoyancy and freedom, and indeed of gaiety of spirit takes the place of the old jaded mental position. It is the pouring in of new wine, but the bottles must also be new or they will burst, and this is exactly what Mr. Alexander's treatment does. It creates the new bottles and then the new wine can be poured in, freely and fully.

Rev. W. Pennyman MA

The case history with which I am most familiar is my own, so I will start with myself:

It all started one cold, dark evening in January. I was driving my car along an unlit street in Bristol, England: all of a sudden the two inner wheels of the car had left the road and I travelled for quite a few yards at an angle of 45 degrees, after which I landed with a large bump. I was shocked and stunned, not knowing quite what had happened. I had, in fact, driven over a two-foot high pile of scaffold boards, which had been concealed in the darkness.

After a few days I started to develop backache in the lumbar region so acute that I could hardly move. After a month or two the backache had eased, leaving me with sciatica. I went to my doctor who gave me some pain-killers and told me to rest. After being off work (I worked as a driving instructor and sitting was the worst position to be in) for six weeks the pain was no better, if anything it was worse. I was then put on a waiting list to see the back specialist at the local hospital. After many X-rays and various examinations no one was any the wiser as to why I still had the pain.

Nearly a year had elapsed. I was then referred to another specialist, but to no avail. All this time the sciatica persisted. After another six months I was asked to attend the physio-therapy department for treatment; this did bring some relief, but only for a matter of hours.

At this point in the proceedings I was offered a choice; either I would have to undergo a major operation, knowing that the surgeon did not know what was wrong, or I could go into a residential physiotherapy hospital, Farnhan Park, one of the largest of its kind in England. After a week of intensive treatment at Farnham Park my back was hurting more than ever, so I discharged myself without any hope of a cure.

After a short while I started to see an osteopath, which really helped to relieve the pain, but again only temporarily. He did, however, suggest I try the Alexander Technique.

I had heard of it by name, but never quite knew what it was. Within a short period of time I had learnt how to help myself; the pain gradually began to abate spontaneously, a great relief after nearly three years of constant discomfort. Within a month of starting my lessons I was able to stop taking the pain-killers that had become part and parcel of my life.

My mental and emotional states also improved, because there is nothing like continuous pain to make one feel depressed and worn out.

Patsy Spiers: Age: 49   Occupation: Midwife

Patsy started coming to a day class with twelve others. She was suffering from a stiff neck which gave her pain whenever she turned her head. She was also prone to frequent and severe migraine headaches, and she had a wheezy chest which had led to her first asthma attack which worried her greatly.

After attending the class for two terms, including a little individual work, she reported:

The Alexander Technique, which is a way of allowing the body and mind to work together in order to avoid muscular tension, has constantly helped me to be calmer in stressful situations. It has also aided me to be more relaxed whilst driving. The stiff and painful neck has returned to normal, my wheeziness has improved greatly with no sign of the asthma returning, and my migraines are far less frequent and not nearly so intense. Although I feel I have a long way to go, I'm a lot more aware of myself, so whenever I get twinges of pain I adjust accordingly and the pain immediately eases. Although I still suffer from headaches, it takes a lot more physical and mental stress before it manifests.

Pat Vince: Age: 58   Occupation: Bank clerk

When Pat came to me in the autumn of 1989 she was suffering from osteoarthritis of the neck and spine with accompanying raised blood pressure. She had tried everything, including osteopaths, chiropractors, pysiotherapy, traction and, finally, pain-killers which she was taking four times a day, every day. She had this to say about her experience of the Technique:

I knew absolutely nothing about the Alexander Technique and viewed it with a certain amount of scepticism, but I felt I had nothing to lose. I did not hope for very much when I began my Alexander lessons, because of my past experiences. My main aim was for some relief to the back pain that I had had for many years but, having tried many other so-called 'back pain-relief techniques', without much success (some worked for a short while, others not at all or even made the pain worse), I was not too optimistic. I was also interested in the possible help for tension, worry and lowering my blood pressure which had lately begun to rise and which concerned me greatly.

Now nearly a year later, attending one class a week and one weekend workshop, and no private lessons, I have been transformed by the Technique. I have found great relief from back pain, my tension and worry is very much reduced, and my doctor has given up even taking my blood pressure.

I have become much more aware of the workings of my body and have begun to use it in a way that is much more economical. I become aware when parts of my body become tense and, more importantly, I know now how to 'relax' them, and when my body is saying that it has had enough I am able to leave things till tomorrow instead of insisting that they have to be done today. This naturally leads to a lessening of tension in the body. The lessons on the causes and remedies of worry were most beneficial and the psychology of using your mind in order to create a change in the body, which came through in most of the classes, helped to reduce the constant tensions in my mind, with the result that I am a much less tense person and a lot of my worries have just vanished.

I have learnt enough about the Alexander Technique to realize that I have much more to learn, and that noticeable change can be a slow process, but I am more than happy with the benefits that I have received so far.

Josie Morton: Age: 67 Occupation: School secretary

Josie was in a great deal of pain when I first met her. Her body was riddled with arthritis. She had aready had one of her hips replaced and the other one was going the same way. She also suffered from arthritis in the wrists, the fingers and the ankles and she was unable to turn her head at all; this was due to a car accident several years before when she had suffered from whiplash.

This is what Josie had to say about her experience of the Alexander Technique:

The reason why I joined the original class was that I had become intrigued by what I had heard and read about the Technique and I thought it might help prevent a second hip operation.

To begin with I found it almost too much to take on board, but it was all extremely thought-provoking and I had to make a decision to put my heart into it or not to bother at all; it would have been pointless just to dip into it now and again. I slowly began to realize that the Alexander Technique not only covers the physical body, but also the mental, the psychological, the emotional and even the spiritual . . . a sort of 'sorcerer's stone'.

It has given me an insight into the way that I behave and that the way that I think definitely affects my actions. Physically, there is a lot more movement in my neck and although I still have the arthritis there is a marked improvement all round. I have confidence that I will not, after all, have to have a further operation. I look forward to the lessons and always feel better immediately, but the difficulty with me lies in trying to maintain my awareness between the lessons, but this is gradually becoming easier. I regard it as a way of living for the future, but what I feel I have learned so far is just the tip of the iceberg.

Patrick Stanton: Age: 35   Occupation: Builder

Patrick had fallen off a ladder over a year and a half ago and had been off work for much of that time. Although the initial injury he had received had healed in a relatively short period of time, he had been left with a pain in his left knee; this was aggravated whenever he put pressure on the joint concerned, as in walking or even just standing.

After having only ten lessons at weekly intervals he had this to say:

I had been in constant pain, since my accident, for nearly two years when I stumbled across the Alexander Technique. I had become withdrawn and at times very depressed which, of course, had repercussions on my family. They were very sympathetic but after a while the tension began to build with ever-increasing rows.

I couldn't go back to work although I had tried several times and socializing was no fun at all. The pain and torment were beginning to take over my life.

After my fourth or fifth lesson I was able to see that it was I who was causing myself the discomfort. I had got into the habit of tensing up my left leg which I probably did, initially, when I had my accident. I couldn't believe it at first that the problem was so simple; in fact I walked out of that lesson without any pain at all . . . the first time for twenty months. The pain did, in fact, return the next day, but this experience had given me hope so I persevered with the lessons and now I am free of the pain for at least 95 per cent of the time. During the process, however, I have learnt so much about myself which I would never have known otherwise. I am deeply grateful to the Technique and to my teacher for the patience that he had.

Val Oatley Age: 62   Occupation: Former ballet dancer

When Val came to me, in October 1989, she had arthritis in both her hands and feet, her shoulders and neck were in pain and she also suffered from chronic sciatica. After completing a course of day classes she had this to say:

By means of the Alexander Technique I have acquired an awareness of where my body is in space which means I am now able to control my muscle tension by means of my brain; this is essential if I was ever to maintain a posture without straining my body unconsciously.

I have discovered a completeness of my mind and body so that it can work as a whole entity, instead of as a jumble of separate limbs, head and torso all working independently of one another. This, of course, relieves a lot of unnecessary muscle tension and teaches me a way of restoring the completeness of the body in a relaxed and coordinated way that had been lost in my early childhood.

Most of my aches and pains have dropped away leaving me able to achieve a balance and poise not only of the body, but of the mind as well.

Yvonne Dartnall Age: 49   Occupation: Owns and runs a hotel

When Yvonne joined my classes she was suffering from tense shoulders and migraines which were very frequent and so intense that all she could do was to lie down while the attacks were present. After attending a regular two-hour class for seven months she wrote:

In my late forties, I was reaching a very difficult period of my life, for no matter what the ailment I was informed by my doctor and friends, 'Don't worry – it's just your age dear. You will just have to put up with it.'

I found this difficult to believe but, before I continue, I will tell you a little about myself. When I was forty I suffered from my very first migraine, I was in bed for five days with it. Before this point in my life I had never really been ill, so you can imagine the disruption within the family. My children and my husband were worried sick because they could all see me lying there in agony without any signs of physical defects.

As time passed the attacks became more and more frequent with three or four attacks each year. At around the age of forty-six the attacks became more intense and, by the time I had reached the age of forty-eight they were a fortnightly affair and almost unbearable. Any visit to the doctor always resulted in a prescribed medication that was ineffective.

So now I was becoming desperate, so I tried an osteopath and was able to get a little relief from minor repositioning of the discs. I was becoming so tense that my head, neck and even my eyes were always so painful. It was then that I decided to help myself, so I went along to the local college and enrolled in what appeared to me to be 'a way to relax' – the Alexander Technique.

That was seven months ago.

My last migraine of any consequence was over four months ago, but I would not be so brash as to say that I have been cured. I can now take precautionary action, however, with the knowledge that I now have, to limit the severity of the attack and even sometimes prevent the attack itself.

Hopefully, in the near future, I will say that I am cured, but I do know that whatever I have learned about myself, through the Alexander Technique, will always be with me in the future and will help me through any other crisis in the time to come.

Learning about our bodies and how they work is obviously very beneficial. It is important to remember, however, that the Alexander Technique is not a treatment or a cure, because you will have to take an active part in the process.

As I have said before, you will be curing yourself.

4

How Does the Alexander Technique Work?

My technique is based on inhibition, the inhibition of undesirable, unwanted responses to stimuli, and hence it is primarily a technique for the development of the control of human reaction.

Frederick Matthias Alexander

THE ALEXANDER TECHNIQUE is a way of heightening awareness of both body and mind. It is based upon two fundamental principles:

1. Inhibition.
2. Direction.

By applying these two principles you will quickly see how unconscious so many of us are as we go about our day-to-day lives.

INHIBITION

We are nature's unique experiment to make the rational intelligence prove sounder than the reflex. Success or failure of this experiment depends on the basic human ability to impose a delay between the stimulus and the response.

Jacob Bronowski

Alexander defined inhibition as the *restraint of direct expression of an instinct*. He realized that, in order to bring about the changes he was seeking, he would first have to inhibit (or stop) his habitual instinctive response to a given stimulus. By checking ourselves a moment before taking action, we give ourselves time to use our reasoning powers in investigating the most efficient and appropriate way of performing such an action. This is a vital step towards having the power to choose freely on every level.

In this way, we see that before the brain can be used as an instrument for ACTION, it first has to be used as an instrument for INACTION. The ability to DELAY (pause) our responses until we are adequately prepared is what is meant by INHIBITION. This moment of pausing before acting has nothing to do with freezing or suppression. Neither is it about performing actions slowly.

Instinctive Inhibition

The best examples of natural and instinctive inhibition are shown in the cat family. Even the domestic cat, when it first sees a mouse, does not immediately rush to capture its prey; instead, it waits until the appropriate moment so as to achieve the highest chance of success.

A cat inhibits the desire to spring prematurely and controls to a deliberate end its eagerness for the instant gratification of a natural appetite.

Frederick Matthias Alexander

It is an interesting fact that, while being fine examples of inhibition and control, cats are also amongst the fastest creatures on earth.

The cat's ability to pause is instinctual – in other words, it is an automatic function of the subconscious brain. Man, by contrast, has the potential to make this ability subject to conscious control, and it is this very difference which clearly divides him from the animal world.

Alexander firmly believed that man has to delay his instantaneous response to the many stimuli that he is bombarded with each day if he is ever to cope with his rapidly changing environment. As man's direct dependence on his body to attain subsistence has decreased, his instinct has become increasingly unreliable; it has become necessary, through the use of inhibition, to employ his conscious powers to fill the gap that has been left behind by its deterioration.

Conscious Inhibition

If we are ever to change our habitual response to given stimuli we have to make a conscious decision to refuse to act in old automatic and unconscious patterns; that is, to say 'no' to ingrained habits.

By inhibiting our initial instinctive action we have the choice to make entirely different decisions. Inhibition is an essential and integral step when practising the Technique. Alexander summarized it thus:

Boiled down, it all comes to inhibiting a particular reaction to a given stimulus – but no one will see it that way. They will see it as getting in and out of a chair the right way. It is nothing of the kind. It is that a pupil decides what he will, or will not, consent to do.

There are many old sayings and proverbs that point to the wisdom of thought before action, such as 'look before you leap', 'more haste, less speed', 'second thoughts are best', and so on.

If you are able to prevent yourself from performing actions that put undue strain on your body then you are already halfway to your goal. To refrain from an action is as much an act as actually performing it because, in both cases, the nervous system is employed. It is also possible, and indeed desirable, to inhibit any unwanted habits and tendencies, not only before an action takes place but also *during* any given activity.

There are many ways of practising this in daily life. For example, every time the telephone or doorbell rings, pause for two seconds before answering (you may find this simple exercise harder than it might seem!); or, if you find yourself in a heated discussion or argument, count from ten to one before responding. (As well as being a useful exercise in inhibition this will also give you time to think about what you really want to convey.)

Try placing a chair in front of a mirror. Stand up and sit down in your normal way and see if you can notice any habitual tendencies (anything which occurs every time). Do not worry if you cannot observe these. Then repeat the above but, this time, pause for a moment before any action while you consciously refuse to sit down or stand up in your normal way. Soon you will realize that there are many different ways of doing the same action. Can you notice any differences between the first and second ways of performing this action?

You may need to carry out the above exercises a few times before you get any results.

THE PRIMARY CONTROL

One of the most noticeable tendencies that Alexander observed in himself was the constant tightening of his neck muscles, the sterno-cleido-mastoid and trapezius. Initially, he presumed that this phenomenon was merely a personal idiosyncrasy, but later observations showed that this was not the case at all: the tensing-up of neck muscles is practically universal. The habit invariably leads to a pulling back of the head onto the spine, thus compressing the intervertebral discs and shortening the structure. This constant pressure on the spine is the main reason for people 'shrinking' with age.

The pulling back of the head also interferes dramatically with what Alexander called the 'Primary Control'. This is simply a term which describes the relationship of the head, neck and back to one another which acts like the major reflex and has the power to control all the other reflexes so as to direct the body in a coordinated and balanced way. It is called 'primary' because all the other reflexes throughout the body are affected by it.

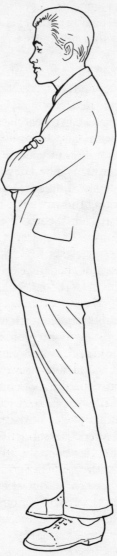

Fig. 4.   A common standing position – the back is hollowed,
with the hips and stomach thrown forward, causing fatigue and
bad internal pressures

Experimental Evidence

A professor of pharmacology, Rudolph Magnus, was very interested in exploring the role that physiological mechanisms play in affecting mental and emotional well-being. Magnus was struck by the central function of the reflexes that govern the position of an animal's head in relation to the rest of its body and to its environment. Working with colleagues at the University of Utrecht, he performed many experiments to find out the nature and function of postural reflexes throughout the body. He wrote over 300 papers on the subject; these pointed to the head-neck reflexes being the central controlling mechanism responsible for orienting the animal to his environment, both in assuming a posture for a particular purpose and also in restoring the animal to a resting posture after an action.

Magnus' experiments, which took place around 1925, only confirmed what Alexander had discovered in himself a quarter of a century earlier. It was found that in all animals the mechanism of the body is set up in such a way that the head leads a movement and the body then follows. In retrospect this seems to be an obvious statement because four of the senses are located in the head and, if we follow our senses as we are designed to, then our head will automatically lead the way.

This phenomenon naturally occurs in all animals with the exception of man whose head is being constantly thrown back when a movement takes place.

A simple exercise can demonstrate this excess tension in the neck muscles: sit in a chair and place either hand on the back of the neck so that the two middle fingers just meet in the middle of the neck at the base of the skull. Stand up, then sit down again, focusing your attention on your hands to detect any pulling back of the head. If you repeat this a few times, you may well notice more tension on the second or third occasion.

Implications of Interfering with the Primary Control

If we are habitually pulling back our heads, so as to interfere

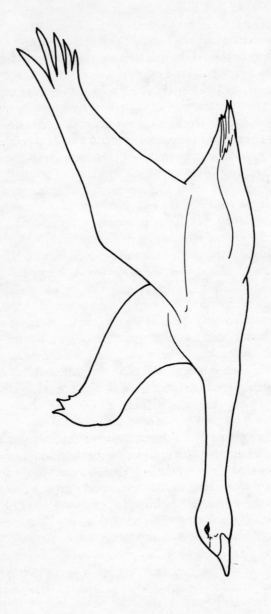

Fig. 5. In all animals the head is designed to lead the movement; the body will then follow

with the Primary Control, then the implications are very serious indeed. Coordination and balance will be severely affected so much so that we hold ourselves rigid in order to avoid falling over. When we come to move we may actually be working against ourselves.

A clear example of this may be seen in the learner driver who grips the steering wheel so tightly with one hand that he has great difficulty in moving the wheel with the other. As a driving instructor I encountered many people who thought that there was something wrong with the car because the wheel would not move easily.

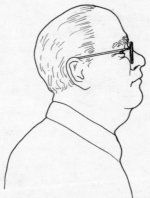

Fig. 6. As we get older the head is constantly being pulled back by excessive muscular tension

The interference with Primary Control builds up gradually, over a period of many years, and because of this most of us are unaware of moving in inefficient, and in many cases harmful, ways. Even when our bodies give us very clear signals that something is wrong, we will hardly ever take responsibility for any problems that we may incur. Most of us, including members of the medical and educational professions, tend to look on pain and illness as natural concomitants of the stresses of living and old age. But such stresses are caused by uncoordinated movements which accelerate the process of ageing.

The other major discovery that Magnus made he called the 'righting reflex'. He noticed that, after an action requiring extra tension (a cat leaping onto a table, for example), a set of 'righting' reflexes comes into play, restoring the body to its normal composed posture. The relationship of the head, neck and back is an essential factor when this righting mechanism is in operation. Therefore it is true to say that, when a person stiffens the neck muscles and pulls back the head, not only is the body's natural coordination being obstructed but it is also being prevented from returning to its natural state of ease and equilibrium.

What a piece of work is a man! How noble in reason! How infinite in faculty! In form and moving how express and admirable! In action how like an angel! In apprehension how like a god! The beauty of the world! The paragon of animals!

Alexander found himself at odds with these famous words of Shakespeare:

'What could be less noble in reason,' he wrote, 'less infinite in faculty, than that man, despite his potentialities, should have fallen into such error in the use of himself, and in this way brought about such a lowering in his standard of functioning that in everything he attempts to accomplish, these harmful conditions tend to become more and more exaggerated. In consequence, how many people are there today of whom it may be said, as regards their use of themselves, 'in form and moving how express and admirable'?

The key to freeing the body to regain its lost dignity lies in inhibiting the unconscious habit of muscle tension; only then may we perform actions in such a way that they become as much a joy to carry out as they are to watch.

SUMMARY

In his own personal development, Alexander became convinced that if he was able to stop doing the 'wrong' thing, then the 'right' thing would automatically happen. But first he had to inhibit his habitual responses. For most of us, the habit of acting without prior thought is very deeply ingrained and, consequently, is not an easy one to 'undo'. Neither is it immediately obvious to us how important it is to inhibit our automatic responses. Inhibition is quite different from suppressing one's own natural responses, although this is how it is often interpreted. Spontaneity is by no means sacrificed by 'inhibition' – the cat, spontaneous and graceful in action and yet perfectly in control of its responses, is a wonderful example of what can be achieved this way.

DIRECTIONS

You come to learn to inhibit and to direct your activity. You learn, first, to inhibit the habitual reaction to certain classes of stimuli, and, second, to direct yourself consciously in such a way as to affect certain muscular pulls, which processes bring about a new reaction to these stimuli.

F.M. Alexander

During his years of experimentation, Alexander was led to a long consideration of the whole question of direction. He asked himself, 'What is the direction upon which I have been depending?', and realized that he had been relying on a sense of what seemed 'natural' and 'right' to govern his actions. Alexander's research had proved these sensory feelings to be unreliable guides and he therefore sought to formulate instructions or orders to himself to replace them.

To give directions is *to project messages from the brain to the body's mechanisms and conduct the energy necessary for the use of these mechanisms.*

You can direct specific parts of the body – for example, you can think of your fingers lengthening – and you can direct your whole body – by thinking of your whole structure lengthening. You can also direct your body through space by consciously

51

deciding where you are going to, and how you are going to get there.

Main Directions

Alexander realized that the root cause of many problems was the over-tightening of the neck muscles, causing an interference with the Primary Control and so throwing the whole body out of balance. The first and most important step, therefore, was to give the orders to ensure a lessening of tension in the neck area so that the normal functioning of the Primary Control could be restored.

The directions he devised were as follows:

1. Allow the neck to be free so that
2. the head can go forward and upwards in order that
3. the body can lengthen and widen.

These orders may vary slightly from teacher to teacher, so that the first order, for example, might be *think of not stiffening the neck* . . .

Allow the Neck to be Free   The purpose of this instruction is to eliminate the excess tension that is almost always to be found in the muscles of the neck. This is essential if the head is to be free in relation to the rest of the body, so that the Primary Control can perform its natural function. This direction should always be given first because other directions will be relatively fruitless without it.

Allow the Head to Go Forwards and Upwards   The head is balanced in such a way that, when the neck muscles are released, the head goes slightly forward, taking the whole body into movement. This direction, therefore, helps the body's mechanisms in their natural functions. If one thought of the head only going forward, and not upward, it would invariably drop downwards, causing an increase of muscular tension in the neck area. It is important to realize that the head should go forward in relation to the spine – as though

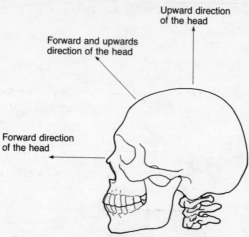

Upward direction
of the head

Forward and upwards
direction of the head

Forward direction
of the head

Fig. 7. Diagram of the head showing the head directions and a combined direction

nodding the head in affirmation. The upward direction of the head is away from the spine and not away from the earth (although these may be the same when the structure is upright).

Allow the Back to Lengthen and Widen   Since the spine shortens when excess muscular tension pulls the head back, it follows that the above direction will encourage a lengthening of the whole structure to the extent that many people who practise the Alexander Technique increase in height by an inch or more. The reason that a widening direction is included is because it is very easy for a narrowing to occur while the lengthening process is taking place.

These three primary directions are, in themselves, very simple and straightforward. They can be quite confusing when first practised as a result of what Alexander called *debauched kinaesthesia*. This confusion is partly due to any difficulty we find in accepting that the solution to a long-standing problem could be so simple; confusion may also arise because, being influenced by the pace of today's world, we presume that we

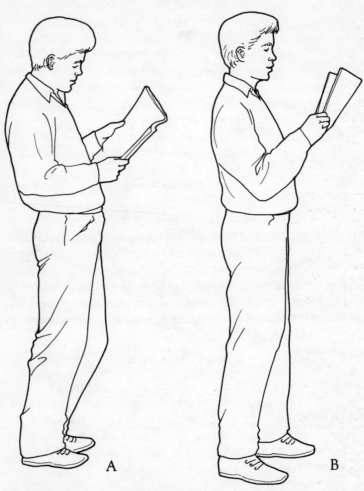

Fig. 8. *Certain standing positions can often cause stress on our bodies without us realizing. In figure A the pelvis is pushed forward so that the man is leaning backwards. This will cause an over-tightening of the entire muscular system. By placing one foot behind the other, as in figure B, the standing position can be very much improved, resulting in our whole structure being much more at ease*

are doing something wrong when we do not achieve immediate results. The answer to this is to be patient and realize that you are changing the habits of a lifetime.

It is strongly advisable that, before you start to give directions, you have at least a few lessons from a trained Alexander teacher to make sure you are on the right track. (A list of teachers can be found in the back of this book.)

Secondary Directions

There are many secondary directions, too numerous to mention here. Whereas the primary directions can be applied universally, the secondary may be applied to certain conditions or ailments. For example, if a person came to me suffering from rounded shoulders I might give him or her an instruction to 'think of your shoulders going away from each other'. Or, if someone came to me with arthritis of the fingers, I might ask him to 'think of your fingers lengthening'.

Here are some examples of secondary directions commonly used in the teaching of the Technique:

When Sitting
* Think of the shoulders going away from each other (for rounded shoulders).
* Think of the sitting bones releasing into the chair (for arched back).
* Think of the feet lengthening and widening (for collapsed arches).
* Think of the shoulders dropping (for hunched shoulders).
* Think of the elbows dropping (for tension in the arms and shoulders).
* Think of the hands lengthening and widening (for arthritis).
* Think about not arching the back (for arched back).
* Think of the ribcage dropping (for breathing problems).

When Standing   Most of the above apply, plus:
* Think of a lengthening between feet and head (general).

* Think of letting your weight go evenly through the soles of your feet (for balance).
* Think of not bracing the knees back (for excess tension in the legs).
* Think of not pushing the hips forward (for backache).
* Think of lengthening between the navel and the upper part of the chest (for depression).

When Walking   Many of the above apply.

There are many more directions to suit an individual's needs, but the primary directions *always* precede any secondary direction that may be given. The word *allow* may often be substituted for the words *think of* – try both and note the different effects on the body. The most important factor to remember is to think or allow. Never try to DO anything. This always increases muscular tension which is the very opposite of what you are trying to achieve.

Right Direction

The last type of direction is that of directing your body as a whole entity – 'What is the direction that I am going in?'

Many people associate the Alexander Technique with putting particular parts of the body into certain positions which they then hold in place thinking that this is improved posture. But holding these positions creates muscular tension which, ultimately, replaces one habit with another. The Technique sets out to do precisely the opposite of this, namely, that parts of the body remain free from other parts no matter what position you may adopt. This, of course, is essential for free movement to take place.

Alexander was adamant that there was no such thing as a right position, but there was a right direction.

There are many more directions than the ones I have men-tioned and these may be used according to one's own particular habit. There is, however, one universal habit which involves tightening the neck muscles and this will invariably interfere with the Primary Control and, subsequently, with all the other muscles and reflexes in the body. By thinking of the main directions you will allow the Primary Control to work as it should and this, in turn, will naturally organize all the other reflexes and muscles.

Directions, along with inhibition, forms the backbone of the Alexander Technique. By applying these two principles, you will be able to change your old habitual ways of moving and will, in turn, experience a new and improved use of yourself. Consequently, you will slowly be able to eliminate many ailments that have been caused by long-standing patterns of misuse.

5

Helping Ourselves

It is essential that the peoples of civilization should comprehend the value of their inheritance. That outcome of the long process of evolution which will enable them to govern the uses of their own physical mechanisms. By and through consciousness and the application of a reasoning intelligence, man may rise above the powers of all disease and physical disabilities. This triumph is not to be won in sleep, in trance, in submission, in paralysis, or in anaesthesia, but in a clear, open-eyed, reasoning, deliberate consciousness by mankind.

Frederick Matthias Alexander

THE FIRST QUESTION that everyone asks, when sick, is 'What can I do to help myself?' But really this is the wrong question because most of us are doing far too much already. Maybe the question, 'What is it that I have to undo in order to help myself?' is more appropriate when it comes to the Alexander Technique. In order to answer this we first have to become aware of ourselves and how we go about certain actions. We are all taught from a very early age that if we are going to get anywhere in this life, we have got to make effort. To a point that is true, but often that effort results in an over-exertion of ourselves which can leave us fatigued and exhausted.

At first, being so aware of ourselves may seem very strange; this is because we are not used to it. For the most part people move around the planet completely ignorant of the way they move. Even when we do become more aware, how do we know whether what we are doing is 'right' or 'wrong'? Well, no one movement can be said to be wrong, it is the repetition of a movement that begins to put a strain upon the body. So the more conscious we are the less likely it is that our activities become habitual.

Look at children while they are walking. Sometimes they will walk fast, even running from place to place, and then they will skip or hop, and the next moment they will be walking quite slowly (much to their mothers' annoyance). The size of their steps is also very varied. Yet you can often recognize an adult by the way he or she walks. This is because our movements slowly become stereotyped as life goes on and we tend to move in a way that feels 'right' to us. We never question that feeling, we just go on in our habitual ways until we are stopped short by one of the many illnesses that afflict our civilization today. Even then, we rarely realize that many ailments are directly, or indirectly, brought about by the way in which we think and move.

Alexander said that everyone wants to be right but no one stops to think whether their idea of right is in fact right. He called this very common human condition 'our faulty sensory perception'.

FAULTY SENSORY PERCEPTION

The main problem that people encounter as they begin to practise the Alexander Technique is the same as Alexander experienced when he was developing his Technique, that is, an unreliable sensory feedback mechanism. In other words, the actions that we intend to do may be completely different from those that we actually carry out. As you will remember in Chapter 2, Alexander discovered that the cause of his vocal problem was that he was pulling his head back and down onto his spine. Until he saw this phenomenon in the mirror, he had been completely unaware of it. His sensory feedback had not informed him that this was happening even though the tension needed to throw his head back had been tremendous.

Even when he tried to put this matter right, by putting his head forward and up, he was faced with an even greater difficulty because he saw again from the mirror that he was increasing the tension and pulling his head back even further. He could hardly believe his eyes and it was then he knew that he was unable to rely on his sensory feelings (the kinaesthetic sense). In the same way we are all under the same delusions in one form or another.

If this is the case we may be standing, sitting or walking in a way that is putting enormous stresses on our structure without us even being aware of it at all. The body is by nature very resilient and it is only years later that the symptoms of misuse emerge. Often the seeds of future ill-health are already sown by the age of twenty only to arise many years later.

As an example of unreliable sensory feeling try closing your eyes and, using your senses and feelings only place your feet so that they are twelve inches apart, parallel with each other. Now open your eyes and see whether the feet are, indeed, parallel and if they are a foot apart. Most people will see that what they feel and the reality of what occurs are two totally different things. Now, with your eyes open, place your feet parallel and nine people out of ten will feel that their feet are pointing inwards. I must point out that this is not the correct way to stand, it is merely an exercise to demonstrate that we cannot rely upon our feelings alone to inform us about what we are doing to ourselves. In all his years of teaching, Alexander did not come across anyone that was not afflicted by the same problem. So you can see that, without professional help, we can make our problems worse, even with the best of intentions. One may say that, if Alexander improved the way he used himself, then anyone can do the same thing. This is true, but do not forget that he spent many hours a day thinking about his problem over seven years. Most of us do not have that sort of time to spare. Alexander's method was brought about by his unique way of thinking which made him the genius that he was. And the benefits that he discovered are now available to us.

AWARENESS

The only measure that we can take to help ourselves is to become more aware of how we go about simple, mundane actions. This will help to bring our minds back into the present more often. Even just being more conscious will help you to perform many actions with greater ease and efficiency of movement.

If you notice a particular position that causes discomfort or pain, such as sitting or standing for long periods, then you do as Alexander did and use a mirror to help you detect the source of your problem. As you can see from the figure on the page opposite the man thinks that he is standing up straight when anyone can see, at a glance, that he is leaning backwards from the waist. This, if allowed to continue, would cause chronic back pain in later life. Any one of us could be under the same sort of misapprehension without even realizing it. A mirror can often be an invaluable tool to help us to become more aware.

At first any new way of being is bound to feel strange, even unnatural, because we have become so used to moving in habitual ways. This strangeness will very quickly pass in the same way as a capped tooth or new filling feels peculiar after a visit to the dentist yet, after a couple of days, we do not even notice it any more. In the same way, when a teacher adjusts you into an upright position you will probably feel as though you are about to fall over in a forwards direction. This feeling will soon pass, however, and you will be left with a sense of poise and balance that had been long forgotten.

After having some Alexander lessons, you will begin to understand the principles of 'inhibition' and 'direction'. Soon you will find that you are taking more time to act, instead of reacting with an habitual response. If there is one factor that really will make a difference to your life, it will be applying inhibition before carrying out any actions. At first it is not easy

61

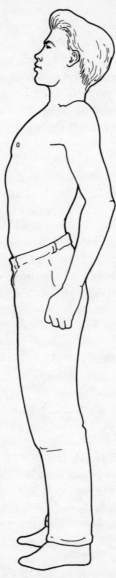

Fig. 9. A clear example of faulty sensory perception. The man thinks he is standing up straight when he is clearly bow-shaped

. . . we usually find that we have completed the task at hand and then we remember that we have not stopped to think first. This will get easier with practice.

You could start from today. Next time the phone rings or there is a knock on the door, just pause for a moment instead of reacting immediately. The level of stress in your body will very soon go down, especially if you are one of those millions of people who rush around every day trying to beat deadline after deadline.

Many people will say that they do not have the time to pause before acting, but this is a false economy; if you do not pause then nature has ways of making you stop through illness. As one of my pupils pointed out – there are a lot of moments wasted when lying on your back for three months. He was only twenty-six and had just recovered from a slipped disc.

A question to ask yourself is this: 'What is more important, the job that I am doing or myself?' We sometimes lose all perspective of what really is important in this life. Alexander realized that the right thing to do would be the last thing that we would think of doing, if left to ourselves.

Try the following movements to increase awareness and help yourself.

Standing

If you have to stand for a while at work or in a queue, it would be helpful to have one leg behind the other with the feet at about 45 degrees to each other. The weight of the body should chiefly rest on the rear leg. In this way the hips are prevented from being pushed forward and therefore are able to support the torso more effectively, thus reducing any excess muscle strain. This will be especially helpful to those who suffer from lower back pain.

Be aware of your feet and where the body weight is being placed. Can you feel more weight on your toes or your heels? Is more weight thrown onto the inside or outside of each foot?

You can often answer these questions by closely examining an old pair of shoes to see the area of most wear.

There are three points of balance on the feet:

1. The heel.
2. The ball of the foot.
3. A point just below the big toe.

All three points should be in contact with the ground if we are to have the maximum stability, essential with such an inherently unstable structure. (We are, in fact, 206 bones piled on top of one another, with the head weighing over a stone delicately balanced on the top.)

Any photographer will tell you that a tripod is necessary in order for the camera on top to remain stable. In the same way all three points need to have equal weight going through them in order to maintain balance and coordination without placing an undue strain upon muscles and joints.

Having said that it is important to point out that there is no one correct standing position. Alexander wrote as far back as 1910:

The Question is not one of correct position, but of correct co-ordination (i.e. of the muscular mechanisms concerned). Moreover, anyone who has acquired the power of co-ordinating correctly, can readjust the parts of his body to meet the requirements of almost any position, while always commanding adequate and correct movements of the respiratory apparatus. Continual readjustments of the parts of the body without undue physical tension is most beneficial as it promotes a high standard of health and long life.

Sitting

It is never a good idea to sit for long periods but, if this is essential, get up from time to time in order to move the body. If you do not do this the muscles may become fixed in a shortened state, putting a strain on joints and various internal organs.

The soles of the feet should be in contact with the ground

because receptors in the feet directly activate the postural muscles throughout the torso. If these are not activated, by having the legs stretched out in front, for example, then you will end up sitting in a slumped manner. This will, of course, affect the breathing and other vital functions of the body.

It might be useful at this point to discuss muscles. There are two types of muscles in the body; these total 650 in number and are known as voluntary muscles and involuntary muscles or postural muscles.

Voluntary Muscles   The voluntary muscles are nearly always attached to the bones of the skeleton and their function is to move parts of the body when we so wish. They always work in pairs, one muscle shortens while its counterpart lengthens, thus moving the bones to which they are attached. At will we can make even the minutest of movements. Muscles can tire, however, after a short time.

Involuntary Muscles   The postural muscles, on the other hand, cannot be used at will. They work when they are triggered by numerous reflexes situated throughout the body. These muscles have the function of keeping us upright against the ever-present force of gravity; they have the advantage of never tiring as they need to work for long periods at a time.

If the body is used in an uncoordinated fashion some of the reflexes are not triggered and, therefore, do not activate the postural muscles. We then start to use our voluntary muscles for support – something for which they were not designed. As a result, we feel very tired after a comparatively short time.

The voluntary muscles will, in turn, contract for long periods and, over the years, become shorter and shorter. This is why, as people get older, they may decrease dramatically in height. People who have Alexander lessons, on the other hand, may gain height because the postural muscles start to work again and the other muscles are allowed to lengthen.

There are also chairs that you can buy, designed by a chiropractor, which are intended to put less strain on the body when sitting. Full information about these chairs can be found towards the back of this book.

Walking

The main factor to remember about walking is to be aware of as much of your environment as possible. It is easy to walk down the road and to be thinking of something else completely. Without us noticing, this will affect our whole balance and coordination. This is because 40 per cent of all the information that is taken in through the eyes is for balance alone. You can prove this for yourself: stand with one leg off the ground so that you are balanced on one leg, and then just close your eyes. Within a few moments you will start to lose your balance. So, if you are not aware of your environment and purposeful in your movements you may be off balance; this will cause many of your muscles needlessly to work harder.

If you look at a small child's eyes, they are always looking in the direction in which they are moving. Sadly, this is not the case with most adults.

Picking up Objects

These days many people know that they should bend their knees when they bend down to pick up an object, but this is only half the story. The other half is that the hips have to bend also, as we can see from the picture of the child on the page opposite. This will keep the whole body in perfect equilibrium and make the action of picking up an object into a comparatively simple activity. What so many people still do is bend from the waist while keeping their legs straight. The result is that they will be using their back muscles, instead of their huge thigh muscles which are much better equipped to do the job. When you do not bend your knees then the back muscles have to support and pick up the weight of your torso, arms and head (70 per cent of your body weight), as well as the object you are carrying.

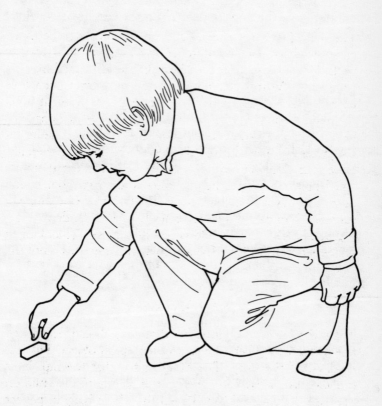

Fig. 10. *The ease of movement shown by a child when picking up an object. Note how the whole body is nicely balanced*

Many back injuries happen this way. The main reason why people act in this manner is to save a few seconds – a high price to pay.

It is interesting to watch professional weight lifters because they always use the thigh muscles to lift the very heavy weights – they have to.

Getting Up from a Chair

Most people expend tremendous amounts of energy when performing this simple activity. This is because they try to get up before their body weight is over their feet. It is much easier to lean further forward before attempting to rise or, if this is not possible, try bringing the feet back so they are almost under the body.

When you have to get up from a settee, it will take less effort if you first come to the edge of it before attempting to stand.

Another very common action is pushing down on the legs to propel the body upwards. But pushing down on the legs stops them from straightening; the legs will then have to work five times harder in order to compensate.

Sitting Down

This action often misuses the body. You can see for yourself that a great many of us fall backwards into our chairs. Whenever the body falls backwards a reflex in the neck (the fear reflex) is triggered: this causes the head to be pulled back onto the spine and the shoulders to be hunched. The reflex protects the very sensitive area at the bottom of the skull and, because it works by reflex, we cannot have conscious control over it. If it is stimulated every time we sit down then tremendous tensions will build up over the years; these will give rise to neck and back problems, and will also be responsible for many headaches and migraines. All you need to do to avoid this reflex is to bend your hips and knees so that your body is balanced until you reach the chair.

Leaning Forward When Sitting

This is a common activity that we all do when writing, typing and eating. To lean forward we usually shorten the front of the torso which will again affect our breathing and all the internal organs. It is far better to lean forward from the hip joints, thus maintaining a lengthening of the entire structure.

All these tips can be very useful in relieving some of the stress that we put on ourselves unwittingly. They are, however, just the tip of the iceberg. An understanding of how we are designed to move in this world is essential if we are to correct our detrimental habits, the source of much pain and discomfort. As we learn to give ourselves more time to pause before activity, we will slowly become more and more aware of the warning signals that our body gives us when it is under stress. In the past most of us have been unaware of these signs and that is why our body ceases to function normally. Our body is very resilient and it is only after years and years of mistreatment that it finally says, 'I can't stand this any more.'

The idea of inhibition may seem easy to apply but, in my experience, this is not the case. It goes against the very nature of man today. We have been programmed from an early age to rush our activities and are only interested in the end product. The way by which that end is brought about is not given any value, and yet our actions can be so creative in themselves. Just look at a swan landing on water, a whale leaping out of the water, or a child playing on the beach – such beauty just in the movements.

END-GAINING

This is a term that Alexander used to describe the nature of modern man. He blamed our 'end-gaining' nature for all the problems that arise in civilization. A clear example can be seen

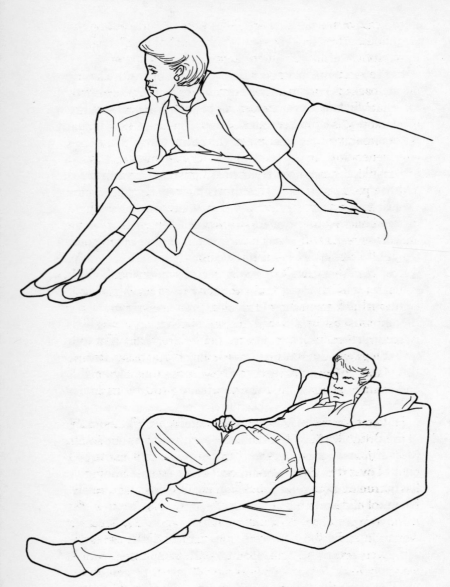

Fig. 11. We may adopt various sitting habits which gradually
distort the body

in the case of the destruction of the ozone layer, causing the greenhouse effect. For the sake of a handful of people making huge profits the entire planet has been put in jeopardy.

In the same way we may stress ourselves at work, causing ulcers, backache and nervous breakdowns in the process, but for what? So that we can make money. Why do we want to make money? So that we can be happy. This way of thinking is not reasonable, yet we carry on in the same way, generation after generation, never learning by our past mistakes. What sets mankind apart from the rest of creation is intelligence and the power of reason. The trouble is we never stop long enough to put them to good use. I once saw a cartoon which pictured hundreds of lemmings throwing themselves off a cliff and drowning in the water below. The caption below read: 'After all, 2000 lemmings can't be wrong.'

Yes, the Alexander Technique is a very useful tool which you can use to help you find the solutions to many physical, emotional and mental problems but, more than that, it has the potential to help us use our intelligence in a way that is constructive both for us and our fellow man. Through technology we have advanced to a point where we can destroy this planet and everything on it. Now is the time to stop this end-gaining mentality and realize what we truly want in our lives.

Dr Peter Macdonald, the president of the Yorkshire branch of the British Medical Association, wrote a letter to the *British Medical Journal* as far back as 1932. In it he said that man's control over the world – steam, explosives, atoms and space – has outrun his power over himself to use that command wisely. No proof of this is needed beyond the tragic conditions of the world today. In time, Alexander will be recognized as a pioneer worker in establishing the conscious control of the use of the self. Every one of his books points to the same thing – unless we apply inhibition in our lives we will never be able to use intelligence in the way it was designed – to assist fulfilment.

6

Practical Exercises

A perfect spine is an all-important factor in preserving those conditions and uses of the human machine which work together for perfect health, yet there are comparatively few people who do not in some form or degree suffer, perhaps quite unconsciously, from excessive spinal curvature.

Frederick Matthias Alexander

ALTHOUGH THERE are no exercises as such when practising the Alexander Technique there are ways of relieving muscular tension in the body. The most common of these is lying on the floor with your head supported on books. The number of books does vary a great deal and your teacher will explain to you exactly how many books are required. If you want to do this for yourself the following method is not quite so accurate, but will give you the general idea.

Book Support

The number of books needed will depend upon your height and the amount of curvature in your spine. To find this out stand, as you would normally, with your heels, buttocks and shoulder blades lightly touching a wall. Get a friend to measure the distance between your head and the wall and add about an inch to the measurement. This will be the height of the books you will need. If you are still not sure, just remember that it is better to have too many books than too few. The number of books may vary as you slowly release the tension in the neck, so

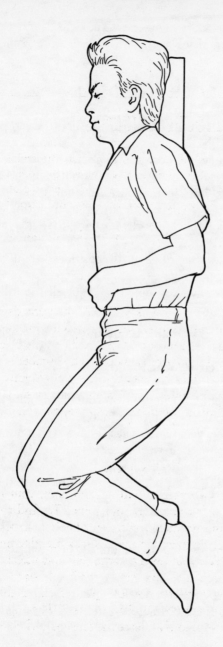

Fig. 12. *The semi-supine position is especially good for lower back pain*

it is useful to recheck the number each month. Be sure that the books used are paperback as this will ensure more comfort.

HOW TO LIE DOWN

Be aware of how you get down to the floor. Get onto all fours and gently roll onto the books. Your Alexander teacher will show you how this can be done with the minimum amount of effort. As you are lying with the books under your head, bring your feet as near to your buttocks as is *comfortably* possible so that your knees are pointing to the ceiling. Have your hands gently resting either side of your navel.

A good length of time to be in this position is about twenty minutes. While you are lying there try to become aware of any tensions in your body. You could ask yourself the following questions:

* Is my back arched so that it is not fully in contact with the ground?
* Are my shoulders hunched so that they are close to my ears?
* Are my shoulder blades not fully in contact with the ground because my shoulders tend to be rounded?
* Do the books feel very hard because I have a tendency to pull my head back onto them with excessive and habitual tension in the muscles of the neck?
* Can I feel one side of my body more in contact with the floor than the other side?
* Can I feel tension in either of my legs? Do they want to fall in or out to the sides?
* Can I feel more pressure on the outside or the inside of my feet?

If the answer to any of these questions is 'Yes', the immediate reaction will be to do something to put matters right. The trouble is that anything you do, no matter what, will nearly always increase the muscular tension and make the situation worse.

According to the Alexander principles, you must try to inhibit any immediate response to your findings and apply conscious thought to help you release tension. In other words you must use your powers of thought alone to let go of any tension that you may feel.

If your back is arched, then think of the back lengthening and widening. After five minutes or so you will begin to see that your back is becoming flatter as it comes more in contact with the floor.

If your shoulders are hunched, think of your shoulders going away from your ears. Very soon you will find that your shoulders are falling away from your ears.

If your shoulders are curving forward towards each other, think of them going away from each other. This should produce a widening of the upper part of the chest.

Do you find that the books are hard underneath your head? If so, think of the head going forward and upwards away from your spine. This will ease the muscular tension in the neck so that the chin drops towards the chest.

If you find that one side of the body is pushing down into the floor, then think of that side of the body releasing away from the floor.

If either leg wants to fall out, then move the foot of that leg away from the other foot. If either leg wants to fall inwards, then place the foot closer to the other foot. This will ease the tension in the legs. Then think of the knees pointing up to the ceiling.

If one side of either foot is more in contact with the ground than the other side, then think of the other side having more contact.

Don't expect any instant changes, as releasing muscular tension takes time. Be patient; there will be changes but nature does take time to work.

Getting Up from the Floor

After about twenty minutes, you should be feeling much more relaxed. Before getting up, pause for a moment or two to work out a less stressful way of rising to your feet. There are many ways of doing this, but one of the best is to roll over onto your stomach and then to go on all fours. Assume a kneeling position and then put one foot in front of the other to come back into a standing position. This may take a little longer than leaping straight up, but it does put less strain on the entire body. This way of rising helps to maintain the length of spine which has been achieved while lying. People with chronic back pain cannot usually get up in any other way.

Anatomical Changes after Lying

The spine, or vertebral column, forms the main supporting structure of the body. It is made up of a number of bones (vertebrae) which are placed one on top of another. They are separated by sacs of fluid known as the inter-vertebral discs. These discs are for shock absorption as well as protection of the bones from rubbing against each other during movement. The discs also absorb fluid in order to increase the spine's length when movement takes place.

In the case of a prolapsed disc (a slipped disc) the vertebrae have been pulled together with a great force arising from muscular tension, so much so that the membrane that encloses the fluid in the disc has burst. This is an extremely painful condition.

The difference in our height changes between the time we get up in the morning and the time we go to bed at night. We can easily lose an inch or more in height as we go about our normal daily activities. This is entirely due to the loss of fluid from discs which are under stress. This loss is regained while we are asleep at night. It is true, however, that 90 per cent of this fluid can be retrieved in only twenty minutes while we are lying horizontally. So if we could lie down for twenty minutes sometime in the afternoon or early evening, then we would lengthen the spine to support us more efficiently for the latter part of the day. We would, therefore, not be so tired at the end of the day and would have more energy to enjoy evening activities. The effect of this is noticeable on people from hotter climates who have siestas; they are able to work into the early hours of the morning without feeling fatigue.

The Decline of Man's Stature with Age

The loss of fluid from inter-vertebral discs is also connected with a slow reduction of one's height over the passage of years.

Have you ever noticed that your parents or grandparents seem to get shorter, even when you have stopped growing?

A scientist by the name of Junghanns discovered, through experimentation, that the size of the inter-vertebral discs does, in fact, diminish as we get older. This is entirely due to excessive muscular tension building up over the years and pulling the bones of the spine closer together, by as much as two or even three inches.

By lying down for twenty minutes each day you can prevent this from happening. You will not only be easing or preventing serious backache, but you will ensure that the discs in the spine are able to maintain their correct shape for longer. This will help you to move in an easier way, putting less strain on your whole structure.

SQUATTING

Exercise programmes often tend to exercise one set of muscles at the expense of another set. But a simple squat can exercise most of the muscles in the body and yet keep it in perfect balance. It is what children do quite naturally and in many under-developed countries people carry on doing it into old age. Because of the many hours of sitting that we do, we lose the ability to squat or even the ability to sit down without falling down.

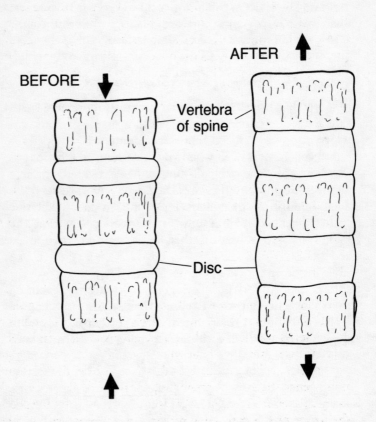

BEFORE

AFTER

Vertebra
of spine

Disc

Fig. 13. *Invertebral discs before and after lying in the semi-supine position*

If you want to know the correct way to squat, then just watch a child of two or three because they are doing it all the time.

When you first start squatting don't overdo it. Start off with small squats, bending your knees and hips just a little. As your legs begin to work so you can go deeper and deeper into the squat. It is so easy to overdo it at first so please be gentle with yourself.

As you improve, start to bring the action into your everyday life, such as when bringing the milk out from the fridge or when picking up the post each morning. It will feel most peculiar at first but, after a couple of weeks, it will feel perfectly normal and your old way will then feel strange.

EYES

Eyes play an important part in the role of body balance and it is important to absorb as much information from the environment as possible. Use your peripheral vision widely when moving from place to place.

Mind-Wandering

Alexander was convinced that many of our tensions are caused by a lack of interest in the present. He referred to this condition as the 'mind-wandering habit'. Very many people spend much of their lives thinking about what is going to happen or what has happened. This, of course, takes us away from the 'here and now'. Since the eyes are an important organ of balance, as well as sight, then it naturally follows that, if we are thinking about the future or the past while walking or standing, rather than playing attention to whatever we are doing, our whole body balance is going to be affected.

For approximately 90 per cent of the time we are thinking about something other than the activity at hand. Sometimes we will be going upstairs to get something but, by the time we are there, we have forgotten what it was that we went for. Many people often walk past their destinations because their minds are thinking about this or that, but not about what they are doing. Have you ever put something of value in a 'safe place', and then forgotten where you put it? I'm sure the answer must be 'yes'. The reason why this happens is that you are thinking about other issues at the time.

The most common statement that drivers make after an accident is, 'I never even saw him coming.' This is because, although we go through the movements of looking, we do not actually see what is there.

So this habit of letting our mind wander can be very dangerous as well as time-wasting and inconvenient.

While giving a pupil a lesson, it is possible to feel the muscles tense in order to maintain balance as he or she begins to lose awareness of the surroundings when 'mind-wandering'. Not being in the present will contribute a great deal to the unhappiness caused by worries and anxieties of modern-day living, because we allow our minds to dwell upon the past which we cannot change and the future which has not yet happened.

In the Present

As children we have a natural ability to experience life from moment to moment, as is also true with animals. We are soon, however, encouraged by society to look to the future for our happiness. Christmas is a good example of this: ten weeks before Christmas arrives, the shops start to fill up with goods which obviously encourage us to dwell on a day that is far ahead in the future. Many of us look forward to that festive season and yet say after the event, 'I am glad that is over.' An interesting fact is that more people commit suicide at Christmas than at any other time. In many cases this is due to great disappointment: if you cannot enjoy yourself at Christmas when can you enjoy yourself?

And what happens on Christmas Day itself? More advertisements on the television, this time about those exotic faraway places which will really make you happy and where you can lie in the sun!

This is just one example of many which encourages all of us to think about the past or the future – but never to be aware of the present. It may be said that we have to plan for the future, and I entirely agree, but most of our thoughts can be best described as nonsense. We have not chosen to think these thoughts, our mind has just started to think them without us being aware of what we are thinking.

We start to lose control of our minds in the same way that muscular tension is often out of our control.

The Alexander Technique is a way of directing our conscious minds in order to be more in the present moment. In this way we have the opportunity to be more in tune with nature and to heighten our awareness of the things around us. This will automatically bring more happiness, contentment and peace into our lives.

PREVENTION IS BETTER THAN CURE

Practising the Alexander Technique is a slow process of examining every area of our lives to find out what it is that is going wrong. By undoing our mistakes at an early stage, before symptoms manifest, we can prevent many of our problems.

It is, however, easy to become anxious about applying the Technique in our day-to-day lives, even though we may have been shown what to do and even though we know that our ordinary sensory perception may be faulty. This anxiety will cause tension which defeats the purpose of the exercise.

If you are patient, however, you will gradually begin to notice changes in the way that you perform actions. These will help the body to perform more efficiently and in a way for which it was designed.

We apply the principle of prevention to other areas of our lives; we regularly visit the dentist even when when there is no pain; or we have fire and burglar alarms installed. Most of us will have our cars regularly serviced as a precaution against mechanical breakdowns and, in industry, there are many rules and regulations to stop accidents ever taking place. Yet we do not apply the same common-sense principles to our own bodies. A little forethought can often save us much pain or discomfort. So many people get backache, for example; most of this would be totally unnecessary if there was a preliminary pause for thought.

If the Alexander Technique was introduced into schools the country could save thousands of millions of pounds each year from the cost of the National Health service, let alone the misery it would save for millions of people. It is not only the patients that suffer, it is also their friends and relatives.

The mounting costs to the Health Service make it apparent that the whole system needs some serious re-thinking. This must be done by people on all levels involved in health-care, including the insurance companies who could save themselves a fortune in claims. The time is also right to give more responsibility to the general public where it rightly belongs; after all, it is your body that is being affected. In order for this to happen it is imperative to educate people in general so that we may have a much greater knowledge of the fundamental causes of both health and ill-health.

To my mind there could be no greater re-education than that offered by the Alexander Technique.

HELPING YOURSELF

You will save yourself much time and trouble if you have a course of lessons from a qualified teacher (all the information you need is in the next chapter). Most of us have the problem of faulty perception or, as Alexander often referred to it, 'debauched kinaesthesia'. Without professional help we can so easily aggravate the problem. Not only have teachers had a very extensive training, they can also be much more objective in seeing the cause of any problem.

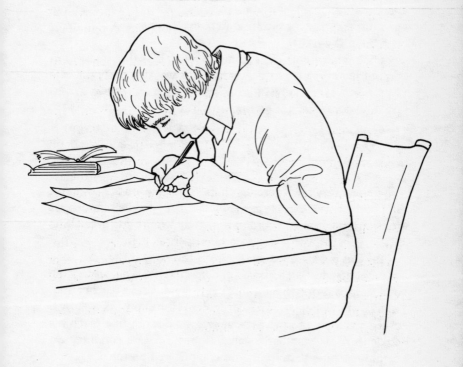

Fig. 14. *Many years of hunching over school work can seriously affect our posture and breathing*

We, on the other hand, will try with added muscular effort to put things right because we will invariably go by what *feels* right. This is what Alexander experienced and is the very reason why it took him so long to sort out the problem with his voice. I would like to point out that when your Alexander teacher talks about 'unreliable feelings' he is talking about sensory feelings and not emotions or intuition (a point that has confused many people in the past).

The main trouble with 'doing it yourself' is that many of us do not have a clue where to start. This was definitely the case with me and, even now, I occasionally have one or two lessons to make sure I am not getting into bad habits.

OTHER EXERCISES

There are very few exercises that do not put undue strain on the body; this strain is caused by the same habits of muscular tension and lack of coordination that we use for everything else (perhaps even more so). Even gentle exercises, such as Yoga, can put tremendous stress on the body if they are done without first dealing with the fundamental issues of end-gaining and faulty sensory perception. A very famous Yoga teacher from India came to England and, after observing many Yoga classes, asked the instructor why it was that he did not first teach his students to sit, stand and walk with balance and coordination before teaching them the more complicated postures.

Walking, running and swimming are the best exercises you can do if you are using yourself in the correct way.

7

Taking It Further

Until one is committed there is hesitancy, the chance to draw back, always ineffectiveness, concerning all acts of Initiative and Creation. There is one elementary truth, the ignorance of which kills countless ideas and splendid plans; and the moment one definitely commits oneself, then Providence moves too. All sorts of things occur to help one that would never have occurred. A whole stream of events issues from the decision, raising in one's favour all manner of unforseen incidents and material assistance which no man could have dreamed would have come his way. Whatever you can do or think you can, begin it. Boldness has Genius, Power and Magic in it. Begin it now.

Goethe

THERE ARE THREE WAYS to learn more about the Alexander Technique.

1. By reading other books.
2. By having Alexander lessons.
3. By attending courses, seminars or workshops.

READING OTHER BOOKS

There are a few informative books on the market today, including four by Alexander himself. A list of these books may be found in Further Reading at the end of this chapter.

85

ALEXANDER TECHNIQUE LESSONS

Anyone who wants to gain the maximum benefit from Alexander lessons should be committed to a course of individual sessions with a qualified teacher. The number of lessons will vary from pupil to pupil, depending on their initial level of balance and coordination. If you have something wrong with your body you must expect between twenty and thirty lessons.

The length of lessons will vary from teacher to teacher, but the shortest will be half an hour and the longest will be an hour.

Cost

This will vary, depending on where you are and how much experience your teacher has had. Lessons will start at around £8.00 and go up to as much as £30.00. If you really cannot afford this payment talk it over with your teacher as most will help out if they possibly can.

Lessons may seen very expensive at first, but the combined total is less than what many people spend on a holiday. What you learn in a lesson will stay with you for the rest of you life.

Finding a Teacher

If you send a stamped addressed envelope to The Society of Teachers of the Alexander Technique (STAT), they will send you a list of teachers in your area. You will find a list of societies for several countries at the end of this chapter. All teachers have had the same training, but styles and personalities can differ greatly. Go by recommendation whenever possible, or have one lesson from three or four teachers. The learning process will be assisted if you feel at ease with your teacher.

Your First Lesson

When you meet your teacher for the first time, tell him, or her, as much as you can about why you decided to have

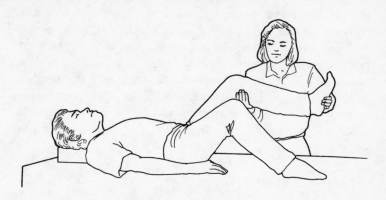

Fig. 15. During an Alexander Lesson, you may be asked to lie on a table while the teacher moves your limbs. When excess tension is found the teacher will ask you to relax specific parts of your body, so that any movement is unrestricted

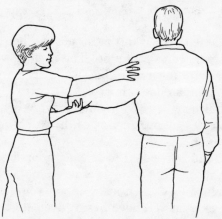

Fig. 16. Due to the stresses and strains of life we can cause a shortening of many of our 650 muscles. This in turn will cause a shortening of our whole structure. In this picture the teacher is helping to reverse the process by lengthening the arm

lessons. If you are in pain (as so many are) be sure you let the teacher know where it hurts and what position of the body causes the most pain. Also tell him how long ago the problem started. If you are in possession of any X-rays, then bring them along with you. Although the Technique does not deal with specific symptoms, it does help the teacher to know any details which might uncover patterns of bodily misuse. Try to be as relaxed as you can – you have made a positive move to help yourself and this should cheer you up.

What to Wear

It is advisable to wear loose, comfortable clothing, although if you have come straight from work this may not be possible and is not essential. You will not be asked to remove any clothing apart from your shoes.

The First Six Lessons

In my experience (and in that of many others) the first few lessons can be quite confusing. The teacher will ask you to lie on a table or to sit on a chair while he gently moves your head and limbs around. He or she is trying to locate areas of tension that may be fixed in your body. When he feels that certain muscles are over-tightened, he will ask you to 'let go' of that tension.

At first you might find it difficult to understand what he is talking about, because most of us are not even aware that these tensions exist. Lesson by lesson you gradually realize the truth of what you have heard. Even then you may find it hard to relax tense muscles as the habits of the muscles are often very ingrained.

Little by little you will start to release any unnecessary tension that may have been stored unknowingly for many years.

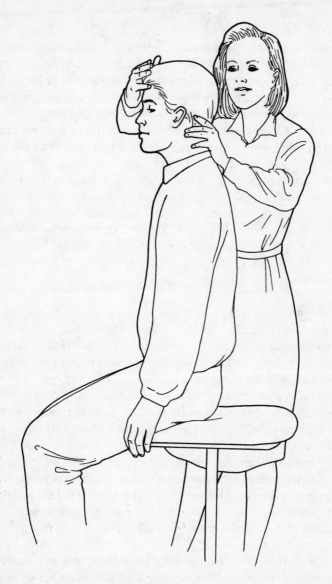

Fig. 17. *The teacher gently alters your position minutely in order to release tension*

Subsequent Lessons

After you have learnt how to release the tension in muscles that have become habitually shortened, your teacher will take you through some ordinary, everyday activities in order to find out why these particular muscles have become over-tightened. Activities, such as walking, standing, sitting or bending, may have to be learned anew. At first, new ways of performing these actions will feel very strange because we have become so used to moving in our own particular way. If left to ourselves, we would never dream of doing anything that does not 'feel right'. After a short while the new way of moving begins to feel less strange and sometimes we cannot understand how we could have moved so clumsily for so many years without realizing it.

Short-term Effects of an Alexander Lesson

Even after your very first lesson, you will probably feel much lighter in yourself. Everything becomes so much easier and some people have an experience akin to walking on air or walking on the moon. This is the result of released muscle tension; gravity affects the body in a different way making it much easier to use. At first, this effect may only last for half an hour but, as you have more lessons, these feelings of lightness, balance and general ease within your body will extend for longer and longer periods. It is then much less effort to carry out many everyday actions.

After the first few lessons it is important to take it easy and not rush around as this may undo the teacher's work and the process will take longer to be effective. It is a good idea not to eat a heavy meal just before having a lesson.

Physical Changes   The day after the lesson you may become aware of tensions in some muscles or you may feel an ache where previously you have had no trouble. Do not worry! This is perfectly normal when the body goes through the physiological changes which are often brought about by the Technique. Not everyone experiences them but they are quite common. I remember, after one lesson, having a sensation of a collar being around my neck which prevented me from turning my head (similar to the kind people have to wear after painful neck injuries). I could, of course, turn my head, I was just beginning to realize that I was constantly holding my head with excessive tension.

Because the muscles are being lengthened, you may experience pain in them. This is similar to the growing pains that we have as children and will soon pass.

Emotional Changes As well as physical changes, you may notice mental or emotional changes. Occasionally, Alexander lessons spark off emotional feelings from childhood – anger, sadness, joy or happiness. Alexander was convinced that every experience is transmitted into muscular tension; as you release the tension you may uncover psychological tensions that have been at the bottom of some physical illnesses.

If any changes take place, either physically, mentally or emotionally, be sure to inform your teacher and he or she will be able to reassure you that it will soon pass.

Long-term Effects of Lessons

The long-term effects can be very varied depending on the individual pupil. If you have come with a particular ache or pain, do not expect it to disappear straight away. What is more likely to happen is that the intensity of the pain will gradually diminish as the weeks go by until, one day, you wake up and realize that it is not there any more.

In the case of reoccurring illnesses, such as migraine or asthma, the attacks usually become less frequent as time goes by; the severity of the illness also diminishes.

Other physical problems, such as clumsiness or bad posture, will slowly start to improve with time. The effects on the body do take a little while to show themselves and sometimes there will be periods when you seem to take three steps forward and two backward. Do not be concerned; everyone feels like that.

The main changes will be seen in the long run when you look back, so it is sometimes useful to have photographs taken of yourself just before, and just after, your course of lessons. These will enable you to see the real changes that have taken place.

Changing Shape   It is often the case that many students grow in height or change their shape in some way during lessons, so it is not a good idea to buy shoes or clothes until nearing the end of the course of lessons. Many of us hold ourselves in the most distorted positions and when tensions are released the changes can be quite dramatic.

It is common for pupils to grow in height as much as an inch and a half; they appear to lose weight at the same time. This is because most of us have a tendency to 'sink' down into our hips so, by allowing a lengthening of the torso, a redistribution of fat tissue takes place and the pupil becomes taller and thinner.

Becoming Peaceful   Mental disorders such as anxiety, depression and insomnia can often be helped since freeing our body from all its stresses and strains will naturally affect the mind. Even if you do not have any problems as such, Alexander lessons will probably help you to feel less irritable and not so worried about life in general. I often hear comments such as, 'Since my husband has been involved with the Alexander Technique he is a much nicer man to live with.'

Most people will gain a greater sense of inner peace – something that is very much lacking in this day and age.

Remember, even if you do not have any specific ailments you will still benefit greatly from a course of lessons, perhaps preventing much pain or discomfort later on in life. This is one of the most important insurance policies you could buy.

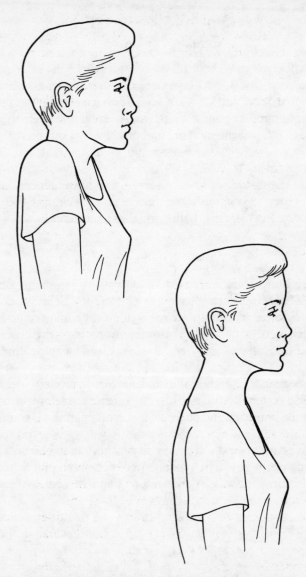

Fig. 18. *Hunched shoulders are very common in our society today. The subject is shown before and after a course of Alexander lessons*

Regularity of Lessons

This will be discussed during your first lesson. Very often your teacher may ask you to come twice a week for two or three weeks and then once a week for a further period which will vary from pupil to pupil. When the Alexander teacher thinks you have grasped the fundamental principles of inhibition and direction, he will ask you to come once a fortnight and then once a month.

After the initial course it is advisable to have an occasional lesson every so often as a reminder and a check that you are not falling into any bad habits without realizing it.

Special Requirements

If there is a certain activity that you wish to improve, please tell your teacher during your first phone call. Some teachers may specialize in certain sports, while others may have had experience of a particular instrument, such as the flute or violin, and therefore may have had similar problems as yourself. Paul Collins, for example, who lives in Somerset, is an Alexander teacher who has explored running and has himself set ten world records for veterans. He, of course, would be an ideal teacher if any sportsmen had running difficulties.

If you cannot find a teacher, who is also an expert in your field, do not worry as any teacher will be able to give you the information that will be required to improve your particular activity.

CHANGE

Alexander once said that people want to change and yet still want to remain the same. By this he meant that many people want to cure a particular problem, or to understand themselves more fully, yet do not want to change their way of moving and, especially, their mental attitudes to life. Most of what we know has been taught to us as children, and, as children, we have adopted ignorance and prejudices which have become more and more fixed as life goes on.

We have to take lessons with an open mind and a humility so that we may find out where we are going wrong. If you are able to say, 'I don't know,' then you will be able to learn the Technique so much the quicker. The reason why some people take a long time to learn the Technique is because it is much simpler than they think.

COURSES, SEMINARS OR WORKSHOPS

In my own experience I have found this medium both economic and a very good way of learning the Technique, especially in the initial stages. At present I run evening and day classes in Devon as well as weekend workshops all over the British Isles. They do not replace individual lessons but in one respect may be even more helpful: seeing another member of the group being shown the basic principles can often make it much clearer to the rest of the group.

To find out about Alexander Technique classes or workshops, ask your local-education authority for details, search your local 'what's on' in the newspaper or look at the noticeboard in your library. If you belong to a group of people or a business firm and would like more information on workshops and seminars, both throughout the British Isles and abroad, then please write to me (address in Useful Addresses section).

I would be more than happy to receive any invitation to take workshops or to give talks on the subject.

I must stress that if you experience much pain, then individual lessons would be more suitable.

TEACHER QUALIFICATIONS

When you initially approach an Alexander teacher, make sure that he or she has undergone a teachers' training course that is recommended by The Society of Alexander Teachers (STAT). A qualified teacher will have undergone a three-year course consisting of twenty hours a week in college as well as home study. Course work is mainly experiential but some basic anatomy and physiology is included. All the teachers on the list that STAT provides are fully qualified.

TRAINING TO BE A TEACHER

When considering whether or not to apply for an Alexander teacher training course you should be aware of the following:

1. Most colleges require a year of continual lessons before applying.
2. There are no government grants to cover either living expenses or college fees.
3. The fees alone amount to between £6000 and £10,000 for the three years, payable at the beginning of each year.
4. Courses usually take students in September although some accept students after Christmas and Easter.
5. Most colleges have a least a year's waiting list.

To train as a teacher is physically, mentally and emotionally taxing. It is not an easy ride, by any means, and you must be sure that it is what you really want to do. Most colleges welcome potential students as observers for a day or two. Addresses of colleges may be found in the Useful Addresses section.

CHAIRS

The wrong sort of chair may be responsible for many of our backaches today. Until quite recently, the Japanese had very few problems with back pain; now it is a problem that is getting rapidly more common. This may well be because our western-type chairs have been introduced into their culture.

Recently I wrote a letter to every car manufacturer throughout the world, offering advice on improving car seats. Not one took me up on my offer to know more! Those that did write back stated that they were very happy with their present designs. Unfortunately, this is not the case with many millions of people whose backache is worse after even a short drive.

There are, however, a few chairs on the market that improve posture while sitting. Some of the best are designed and manufactured by John Gorman who has been very interested in the Alexander Technique for many years. He is an engineer who came to study the spine because of his own back pains. His engineering analysis of the problem brought him to many ideas that were very similar to Alexander's in terms of posture and sitting.

One of his first designs was 'the Simple Working Chair', produced in 1984, which has subsequently given comfort to thousands of people. In his two books on the subject he describes the importance of 'good sitting habits' in maintaining a healthy spine and body; his views are similar to those taught by Alexander himself. Mr Gorman recently trained to become a chiropractor.

The basic principle of his chair is that the knees should be below the pelvis, a quite different principle to the design of most chairs. The usual type of chair puts an enormous strain on the spine, back muscles and many of the internal organs. Anyone sitting down for extensive periods (as we all had to do in our school days) would have to tense many of the body's muscles in order to sit up straight. This, in turn, causes the organs, the bones and, ultimately, the entire system to be under stress.

The forward-tilting chair allows the spine and the postural muscles to support and balance the body naturally. You can easily see the effect by placing a telephone book under each of the rear legs of a ordinary kitchen chair. At first, the sensation may seem strange but, after a few minutes, you will appreciate its comfort. The height and angle of the Gorman chairs can be adjusted to suit the individual. Information on these chairs may be obtained from:

John Gorman
Pelvic Posture Ltd
Oaklands
New Mill Lane
Eversley
Hampshire RG27 ORA

Balance chairs have also attracted a good deal of interest. The forward tilt is admirable but these chairs have a disadvantage: by placing the knees on a pad the feet, with their receptors, are prevented from being placed flat on the floor. Balance chairs are better than conventional chairs but not as beneficial as the Gorman chair.

LAST WORDS

George Orwell once said that, by the time you are forty, you have got the face you deserve. Perhaps the same aphorism could be said of our body. If we are using up to five times the energy that we really need to move, then it is hardly surprising that, after a long day, all we can do is 'collapse in a heap'! We have only one body in this life so it is well worth looking after.

I trust that you have enjoyed this book and that you have found it useful. It was written merely as a simple introduction to the Alexander Technique and I hope it has whetted your appetite to find out more. In the next few pages are listed the branches of The Society of the Alexander Technique throughout the world, from which you can obtain the names and addresses of teachers in your area. Teacher training colleges are also listed, as are books for further reading.

So, I wish you a happy and healthy life and and make no apology for repeating these words of Goethe:

The moment that one definitely commits oneself, then Providence moves too. All sorts of things occur to help one that would never have occurred. A whole stream of events issues from the decision, raising in one's favour all manner of unforseen incidents and material assistance which no man could have dreamed would have come his way. Whatever you can do or think you can, begin it. Boldness has Genius, Power and Magic in it. Begin it now.

Useful Addresses

F OR FURTHER information about week-long courses, weekend workshops, seminars or lectures on the Alexander Technique, both in the United Kingdom and abroad, please contact:

Richard Brennan MSTAT
The Alexander Technique Centre
8 Brooklands
Bridgetown
Totnes
Devon TQ9 5AR
ENGLAND
Tel: (0803) 866010

For a list of teachers in your area please send a stamped addressed envelope to:

United Kingdom

The Society of Teachers of the Alexander Technique
10 London House
266 Fulham Road
London SW10 9EL

Australia

The Australian Society of Teachers of the Alexander Technique
PO Box 529
Milson's Point
NSW 206I

Canada

The Canadian Society of Teachers of the Alexander Technique
PO Box 502
Station E
Montreal
Quebec H2T 3A9

Denmark

DFLAT
Wergelandsalle 2I
DK – 2660
Soborg

The Netherlands

Netherlands Society of Teachers of the Alexander Technique
Max Havelaarlaan 80
II83 H N Amstelveen

Switzerland

SVLAT
Postfach
CH 8032
Zurich

United States of America

NASTAT
PO Box 806
Ansonia Station
New York
NY I0023–9998

Please Note   If you want to find a teacher in a country that is not listed above please write to the London address and they will be pleased to send you a teachers' list that covers the whole world.

TEACHER TRAINING COLLEGES

United Kingdom

London
Centre for the Alexander Technique
46 Stevenage Road
London SW6 6HA

The Centre for Training and Development
142 Thorpedale Road
London N4 3BS

The Constructive Training Centre
18 Lansdowne Road
London W11 3LL

New Alexander School
21 Lyndhurst Road
London NW3 5NX

North London Teachers Training Centre
10 Elmcroft Avenue
London NW11 0RR

The Victoria Training School for the Alexander Technique
50A Belgrave Road
London SW1V 1RH

The West
Bristol Alexander Technique Training School
The Guide Hut
Weston Road
Long Ashton
Bristol BS18 9BJ

The School of Use
Foxhole
Dartington
Totnes, Devon TQ9 6EB

The East
AT Training School
56 St Barnabas Road
Cambridge CB1 2DE

Essex Alexander School
65 Norfolk Road
Ilford
Essex IG3 8LJ

The South
West Sussex Centre for the Alexander Technique
5 Coates Castle
Pulborough
West Sussex HR20 1EV

The Brighton Alexander Technique Centre
57 Beaconsfield Villas
Brighton
East Sussex BN1 6HB

South Midlands
Alexander Re-Education Centre
10 Langdon Avenue
Aylesbury
Buckinghamshire HP21 7UX

The Alexander Technique Training Centre
63 Chalfont Road
Oxford OX2 6TJ

The North
Fellside Alexander School
Lowfellside
Kendel
Cumbria LA9 4NS

Scotland
Alexander Technique Training Course
Madras College, Kilymont,
St Andrews, Fife,
Scotland. KY16 8TB

Australia

Centre for Alexander Technique Studies
245 Broadway
Sydney NSW 2007

Denmark

F.M. Alexander School
Fredriclagade 33V
1310 Copenhagen

Institute for F.M. Alexander Teknik
Solmarkvej 20
8240 Risskov

France

AT Training School
99 Rue de Vaugirard
75006 Paris

Centre de Formation en Technique Alexander
40 Terrace de l'Iris
92400 Courbevoie

Germany

The Alexander Technique Training College
Grillparzerstr
2000 Hamburg 76

AT Training School
Schleissheimersir 173
8000 Munich 40

Training School for the Alexander Technique
Postfach 606
D-78000 Freiburg 1 Br

Holland

Alexander Technick Opleding Nederland
Herengracht 340
1016 CG Amsterdam

Israel

The Alexander Foundation
31 Frug Street
Tel Aviv

AT Training School
13 Israelis Street
Tel Aviv

The Alexander Technique Centre
4 Ayalon Street
Haifa 34336

The Haifa School of the F.M. Alexander Technique
8 Sea Road
Mount Carmel
Haifa

Italy

Centro Italiano Tecnica Alexander
Corso Mastteotti 80
56025 Pontidera
Pisa

Switzerland

AT Training School
Schwelzergasse 38
4054 Basel

AT Training School
Vorderfeldstr 8
CH-8706
Feldmeilen

A.T. Training School
Apollostrasse 8
CH-8032
Zurich

United States of America

The Center for the Alexander Technique
714 Nash Avenue
Menio Park
CA 94025

The Urbana Center for the Alexander Technique
508 West Washington
Urbana
IL 61801

The Alexander Institute of Boston
115 Westbourne Terrace
Brookline
MA 02146

Institute for the Alexander Technique
PO Box 370
Briarcliff Manor
New York
NY 10510

The Virginia School for the Alexander Technique
PO Box 1604
Charlottesville
VA 22902

On completing one of the above courses, you will be issued with a certificate authorized by The Society of Teachers of the Alexander Technique of the appropriate country where you trained. This certificate will be recognized by all the institutions that employ Alexander teachers, that is, most of the major music, drama and adult-education colleges throughout the world.

Further Reading

Alexander, F.M. *Constructive Conscious Control*, Gollancz, 1987.
Man's Supreme Inheritance, Centerline Press, 1988.
The Use of the Self, Gollancz, 1985.
The Universal Constant in Living, Centerline Press, 1986.
These books are of great value; however, they are not easy to read. You may need a dictionary to decipher some of the sentences.

Barlow, W. *The Alexander Principle*, Gollancz, 1973.
Wilfred Barlow was a specialist in the NHS as well as being a teacher of the Technique. This is an interesting book with an emphasis on the medical aspects of the Technique.

Gelb, M. *Body Learning*, Aurum Press, 1981.
An excellent follow-up title to any of the introductory books.

Macdonald, P. *The Alexander Technique as I See It*, Rahula Books, 1989.
A collection of some interesting note-book jottings, of special interest to those already involved in the Technique. Patrick Macdonald was one of the most experienced teachers, having been trained by Alexander himself.

Stevens, C. *Alexander Technique*, Optima, 1987.
This is an easy-to-read book for people who know very little, or nothing, about the Technique.

Westfeldt, L. F. *Matthias Alexander: The Man and His Work*, Centerline Press, 1986.
This is the autobiography of a polio victim who overcame her difficulty in walking and then trained as an Alexander teacher. A very readable book which is quite moving at times.

Index

111